# Cancer

### Causes, Preventions, Cures

---

*What the Food and Beverage Industry does NOT want you to know!*

---

## BY
### DOC WILSON, PhD

# Volcano Erupting at Night

---★★★---

When there is a volcanic eruption, there is massive disruption to those close by the eruption. Similarly, when there is a diagnosis of cancer, there is massive disruption of the patient's life, as well as the lives of their family members, friends, and associates.

The sheer POWER of an erupting volcano represents the POWER that the cancer patient must muster, from within, in order to defeat their disease. The cancer patient must transfer the POWER of the volcano to their inner being so that they increase their internal strength, which defeats the life-threatening enemy – CANCER! If you are this patient, do not let this (CANCER) destroy your entire being – body, soul, and mind!!!

IMAGINATIONPRESS

**HEALTH SMART NO. 1:**

**Your ULTIMATE PROGRAM**

What the Food and Beverage Industry
does NOT want you to know!

Including how to utilize epigenetic principles for better health!

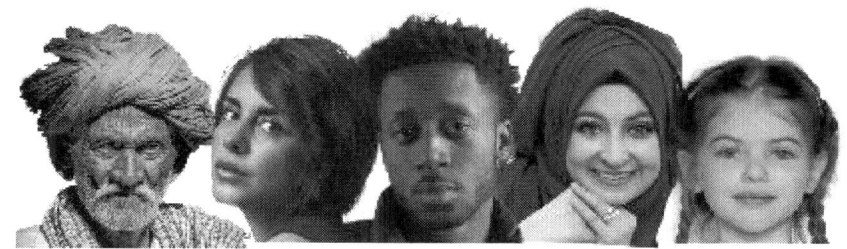

*CANCER DOES NOT DISCRIMINATE*

**DOC WILSON, PhD**

Cancer! Causes, Preventions, Cures © 2021 Doc Wilson

All rights reserved. Printed in the United States of America. No part of this book may be used or reproduced in any manner whatsoever without prior written permission except in the case of quotations embodied in reviews or used for educational purposes.

**Editing by**

Teresa Hamilton

Brandi Dyer

Debbie McGrann

**Researcher**

Tyler LaRoche

**Initial Front Cover Concept design by**

Francis Adams

**Cover Design by**

Brandi Dyer

ISBN 978-17337189-5-0

First Edition: September 4, 2021

# Table OF Contents

Preface ............................................................................................................... 1

Dedications ...................................................................................................... 4

This "Ultimate Program" .............................................................................. 5

SECTION I The WHAT: What Science Concludes ................................ 8

Chapter One   Terror! Cancer: Its Origin and Perspectives ..................... 9

    Cancer: Its Origins ................................................................................. 10

    Cancer in Perspective ............................................................................ 13

References ...................................................................................................... 17

Chapter Two   The 8 Foundational Pillars for Best Health .................... 20

    Notes: ........................................................................................................ 30

    Creating Your Shopping List ............................................................... 31

    Eating 5 or 6 Small Meals a Day ......................................................... 31

    Losing Excess Weight ........................................................................... 31

    Cutting and Washing Food .................................................................. 32

    Raw vs. Cooked ..................................................................................... 32

    Things to Avoid! .................................................................................... 36

    Giving Back ............................................................................................ 36

    Attitude ................................................................................................... 36

    Spirituality .............................................................................................. 37

References .................................................................................................38

Chapter Three   Additional Foundations of Good Health ..................45

Reference ....................................................................................................47

Chapter Four   Various Definitions of "GRADUALLY" and Some Specifics About Making Health Transitions ..................................................48

    For NUTRITION ................................................................................49

    For CARDIO EXERCISE (Interval Training) ...............................49

    For STRENGTH-BUILDING EXERCISE ......................................49

Chapter Five   The Biochemistry of Cancer, and Why Sugar and "Sugar Equivalents" (including "Undeclared Sugars") are So Dangerous to Your Health ..........................................................................50

References ................................................................................................54

Chapter Six   Body Weight and Weight Loss ........................................56

    Some important Notes concerning Interval Training .................60

References ................................................................................................66

Chapter Seven   Strength-Building Exercises ........................................68

    Optimum Order of Exercises ...........................................................72

Chapter Eight   Deep Sleep and the Role of Sunshine ........................73

    The Role of Sunshine ........................................................................75

References ................................................................................................77

Chapter Nine   Stress Reduction and Unexpected Sources of Stress to Your Body ..........................................................................................79

    A Few Tips ..........................................................................................80

References ................................................................................................83

Chapter Ten   Your Mindset ....................................................................85

Reference ................................................................................................................ 87

Chapter Eleven   Avoid Drugs, Smoke, Smoking, and Alcohol! ............................. 88

    The Extra Danger for the Diabetic Who Smokes .................................................. 89

    Alcohol ................................................................................................................ 90

References ............................................................................................................ 92

Chapter Twelve   Type 2 Diabetes and the Increased Risk for Cancers in General ................................................................................................................................ 98

References .......................................................................................................... 101

Chapter Thirteen   Avoiding Noxious Fumes (Gasoline, Vehicle Emissions, Formaldehyde), Asbestos, and Other Environmental Hazards ........................... 105

References .......................................................................................................... 109

Chapter Fourteen   Late Evening Eating Restrictions Eliminate and Reduce Cancer Risks ....................................................................................................... 117

References .......................................................................................................... 119

Chapter Fifteen   Support Groups Online ............................................................ 121

Chapter Sixteen   The Weakest Link Concept ...................................................... 123

Chapter Seventeen   Fitness and Longevity: What Does it REALLY Mean for You? ................................................................................................................... 125

References .......................................................................................................... 127

Chapter Eighteen   Spirituality and Giving Back ................................................. 130

Chapter Ninteen   Miscellany – A Note on Cleanliness ....................................... 132

References .......................................................................................................... 133

Chapter Twenty   The Holy Trinity of Un-Healthy .............................................. 134

SECTION II The WHY: Why Certain Lifestyle Choices are Healthy or Unhealthy ............................................................................................................................ 137

Chapter Twenty-One   Why Being Overweight is ALWAYS Unhealthy ............. 138

References ................................................................................................... 140

Chapter Twenty-Two   Why Being Sedentary is Always Unhealthy ................... 150

References ................................................................................................... 152

Chapter Twenty-Three   Why Not Getting Enough Deep Sleep Virtually Every Night is Always Unhealthy ........................................................................... 160

References ................................................................................................... 162

Chapter Twenty-Four   Why Eating Meat From Mammals is Unhealthy for You ................................................................................................................... 168

References ................................................................................................... 171

Chapter Twenty-Five   Why Not Eating Enough Fruits, Vegetables, and Nuts/Seeds, and Too Much Sugar and Sugar Equivalents, is Always Unhealthy ................................................................................................................... 174

References ................................................................................................... 178

Chapter Twenty-Six   The Truth About Multi-Vitamins and Supplements ....... 180

  Note On African Americans and Other Persons of Color .................... 182

References ................................................................................................... 183

SECTION III   The MORE: If You Desire to Delve Deeper into the Science .......... 186

Chapter Twenty-Seven   How Applying EPIGENETICS Can Reduce Your Risk for Cancer ................................................................................................... 187

References ................................................................................................... 195

Chapter Twenty-Eight   Innovations in Cancer Research ................................. 203

Reference ................................................................................................... 210

Chapter Twenty-Nine   The Relentless Flood of Scientific Articles on Cancer ... 211

Chapter Thirty   Complications Relating to Cancer ........................................ 213

References ............................................................................................................. 215

SECTION IV  CONCLUDING REMARKS AND PERSPECTIVES: Putting It All Together.................................................................................................................. 217

Chapter Thirty-One   Total Health, Total Health, Total Health............................ 218

Reference ................................................................................................................ 222

Chapter Thirty-Two   NO GUARANTEES!!!............................................................ 224

References ............................................................................................................. 227

APPENDIX 1.  Diving Deeper ............................................................................... 231

APPENDIX 2.  A Typically Meal .......................................................................... 233

APPENDIX 3.  Getting your vegetables ................................................................ 235

APPENDIX 4.  CT Scans Can Greatly Increase the Risk for Cancers!................ 237

APPENDIX 5.  CANCER: Fact versus Fiction ...................................................... 238

Reference ................................................................................................................ 240

DOC'S CREDENTIALS ......................................................................................... 241

Prior to making any major changes

in your nutrition or exercise practices,

be sure to consult with your physician.

# Preface

We live in the digital age, which means that, theoretically, we can now more quickly learn about new, groundbreaking research that can help us live longer, healthier, more productive, happier lives. However, I suspect that this ready access to digital information has produced not only a bit of impatience in a lot of people, but also a fair amount of complacency! Only **5 to 10%** of cancers are due to bad genetics; the remaining **90 to 95%** of cancers are due to other causes. In the course of writing this book, I came to realize that many people - including health professionals - are not aware that they can greatly reduce their risk of contracting cancer and or reversing cancer if they get it. This is why I decided to write this book: to "get the word out" to people everywhere! Thus, this book details **what you need to do to greatly <u>reduce your risk for contracting cancer</u>;** or, if you do contract cancer, the lessons from this book **will strongly <u>improve your odds for curing your cancer</u>.**

This concise reference should fit well into your crazy lifestyle because it covers **just the essentials** in all the critical areas for the prevention and reversal of cancer – in a **nutshell format**. This book combines teachings from a variety of disciplines that are highly pertinent to understanding cancer; the impact of, and the relevance of, many of these areas are not appreciated by many physicians – including many oncologists, who you rightfully would expect to keep up on the literature in these areas! Thus, this book bridges that knowledge gap with the intent of improving lives everywhere!

As an example of a vitally important area, this book will help you separate "the wheat from the chaff" in the area of **nutrition.** As you may know all too well, professional nutritionists and dietitians are not in agreement on many important nutritional subjects – which is why you, and millions of others are confused by the conflicting information! (Note: The vast majority of nutritionists and dietitians not only are on *different pages*, but all too often, are also on the *WRONG* pages!)

A second vital area is **exercise.** You may be one of the *silent majority* whose attitude is negative toward exercise. However, **doing at least a reasonable minimum, as is detailed in Chapter 1, will pay _huge_ dividends for your level of health!** As you will discover in these chapters, **you *DO NOT* have to be a gym rat – spending many hours a week – to realize significant results!**

Third, one of the unifying themes of this book is the functioning of your **immune system.** Every day, **every cell in your body is hit with millions of newly formed cancer cells that are seeking to establish a firm toe hold and start growing!** And your immune system has the enormous task of creating antibodies, T-cells, killer cells, etc. to fight off many potential infections and cancers! Regular **application of *every* concept and recommendation in this book will boost the functioning level of your immune system!** My emphasis on *"every* **concept and recommendation"** is not just important; it is <u>CRITICAL</u> because **your health is only as good as** *your weakest link!* (See Chapter 16 for more on this.)

As you read through this book, you may become aware of a fair number of repetitions in such areas as nutrition, exercise, sleep, etc. These areas of repetition reflect the extreme importance of these areas to your best health.

The remaining chapters flesh out the other important areas so that you will have the best tools to fight cancer and be prepared intellectually with **the essentials not only for preventing and reversing cancers, but also for having the best and healthiest body possible!** However, as with all things in life, there are no 100% guarantees; in the domain of cancer, this simply means that your job is **to do everything possible to increase your odds of total success!** Think of this in statistical terms: The larger the number of wise choices that you make, the better your odds will be of preventing and/or reversing cancer!

Doc Wilson, PhD.

# Dedications

I dedicate this book to:

- ❖ My daughter Krista (I cannot imagine a better daughter!)
- ❖ My two grandsons given to me by Krista: Justin and Ryan
- ❖ Marie and Tom Hardy, who have operated "in the background" to help build and promote Imagination Press
- ❖ Francis Adams, the super graphic artist who designed the front and back covers and the layout of this book
- ❖ Teresa Hamilton, my partner, and co-founder of Imagination Press: Her intelligence and perspectives were invaluable in framing and promoting this book
- ❖ My stepmother Joan
- ❖ A special thanks to Eva Havas for her valuable insights

# This "Ultimate Program"

――――――― ★ ★ ★ ―――――――

You may be interested to know that, when you follow the prescriptions of this book, this Ultimate Program will greatly help to prevent and reverse a number of ailments in addition to cancer:

   a. Prevent & reverse **Hypertension** ("High Blood Pressure"), as well as other Cardiovascular issues ranging from **Angina** ("chest pain") to more serious things, such as **Myocardial Infarctions** (MI's or "Heart Attacks")

   b. Prevent & reverse **Strokes** ("bleeding/hemorrhaging into the brain"), and related problems ranging from **Transient Ischemic Attacks** (TIAs or "mini-strokes"), all the way up to **Cerebrovascular Accidents** (CVAs or "full-blown Strokes" as the result of clots shutting off blood flow to a part of the brain), **Peripheral Artery Disease** (PAD), and

   c. **Atherosclerosis** ("hardening of the arteries")

   d. Prevent and reverse **Metabolic Syndrome**

   e. Prevent & reverse **type 2 diabetes**

   f. Decrease the odds of developing many kinds of **Dementia**, including **Alzheimer's Disease**

g. Improve **Mental Health**, including reversing, and reducing the risk for, **Major Depression**

h. **Weight Loss**, including greatly improving long-term success in the "Battle of the Bulge"

i. Reduce unnecessary **Stress**

j. Improve **Overall Health**, including significantly **increasing longevity,** as well as the odds of a healthy, productive, fulfilling, and fun-filled life up to the very end

**NOTE on References:** A fair number of references are cited at the end of each chapter. Some will argue that this citing of many references is overkill. However, I have elected to provide numerous citations to the original, peer-reviewed scientific literature to emphasize two points:

1. **a *lot* of research results** have been published to date, and the many concurring results indicate that the generalizations in this book have a broad, strong foundation; and

2. among cancer specialists, there is general agreement on each of the points that I make on cancer – not just an occasional reference on a given point, or on cancer in just one tissue or one organ, that might well be overturned in a subsequent scientific study; rather, **the strong conclusions and strong generalizations presented in this book often apply to preventing, avoiding, and curing a broad range of types of**

cancers, and of cancers in a wide variety of tissues and organs.

# SECTION I

## The WHAT: What Science Concludes

# Chapter One

# Terror! Cancer: Its Origin and Perspectives

─────────── ★ ★ ★ ───────────

F ew words strike more terror in the heart of a person than a **diagnosis of CANCER!** Numerous thoughts and questions

flood the person's mind, senses, and psyche. For example,

Will I die?

If so, how much longer do I have until I pass away?

How much pain will I experience?

Are there any new treatments that might help reverse my cancer?

Has (or will) my cancer spread to other tissues or organs?

What can I do to extend my time for passing away?

Which members and friends should I tell first?

Are there any **websites or other resources for new, state-of-the -**

art cancer treatments and information?

There are zillions of other questions of this nature that are likely to arise!

## Cancer: Its Origins

Cancer has been around for quite some time – dating back to Egyptian mummies as far back as 3,000 years ago. Bone cancer was one of the earliest forms of cancers found in these mummies.

Hippocrates (460-370 BC), the "Father of Medicine," gave "cancer" its name, based on the "crab-like" ulcers that he had observed in formed tumors. Hippocrates used the terms **carcinos** and **carcinoma** to describe non-ulcer forming and ulcer-forming tumors. In Greek, these words refer to a crab, most likely applied to the disease because the finger-like spreading projections from a cancer looked like the shape of a crab. The Roman physician, Celsus (28-50 BC), later translated the Greek term into **cancer,** the Latin word for crab. Galen (130-200 AD), another Greek physician, used the word **oncos** (Greek for swelling) to describe tumors. Although the crab analogy of Hippocrates and Celsius is still used to describe malignant tumors, Galen's term is now used as a part of the name for cancer specialists: Oncologists.

The Edwin Smith Papyrus, an ancient Egyptian textbook on trauma surgery dating back to 3,000 BC, outlines at least 8 cases of tumors in the breast, which were removed by using a tool called a "fire drill tool." This textbook also noted that there was not a cure for the tumors. The writing says about the disease, "There is no treatment."

Throughout the centuries, various physicians have made more precise analyses of cancer and its spread. In 1713, the Italian doctor Bernardino Ramazzini noticed that cervical cancer was practically nonexistent in nuns, whereas breast cancer was prevalent in nuns. He wondered if these observations were in some way related to their celibate lifestyle. This observation was an important step toward identifying and understanding the importance of hormones (like the changes that come with pregnancy), etc. and <u>sexually-transmitted infections and cancer risk.</u> Thus, he was able to make a connection between the role of hormones and a woman's risk of getting cancer, as well as conclusions about sexually transmitted diseases.

In 1775, Doctor Percival Pott of Saint Bartholomew's Hospital in London noticed an occupational cancer connection between chimney sweepers and cancer of the scrotum when he observed that chimney sweepers often had soot lodged in the skin folds of their scrota that increased their risk of contracting scrotal cancer. This research led to many more studies that identified a number of **occupational carcinogenic exposures**, and led to **public health measures** to reduce a person's cancer risk from their job.

Thomas Venner of London was one of the first to warn about tobacco dangers in his *Via Recta*, published in London in 1620. He wrote that "immoderate use of tobacco hurts the brain and the eye and induces trembling of the limbs and the heart." And 150 years later, in 1761, only a few decades after recreational tobacco became popular in London, John Hill wrote a book entitled *Cautions Against the Immoderate Use of Snuff*. These first observations linking **tobacco and cancer** led to epidemiologic research many years later (in the 1950s and early 1960s) which showed that smoking causes lung cancer and other cancers.

Human beings and other animals have had cancer throughout recorded history; so, it is no surprise that many people have written about cancer. As noted above, some of the earliest evidence of cancer has been found among fossilized bone tumors in human mummies from ancient Egypt, and in ancient manuscripts. Also, growths suggestive of the bone cancer known as **osteosarcoma** have been seen in Egyptian mummies. Furthermore, bony skull destruction as a result of cancer has been observed in ancient bones of the head and neck of skeletons.

Today, cancer is the second leading cause of death in the United States after heart disease. We now know that most people contract cancer due to a number of adverse conditions in the environment (smoking, pollution, etc.) and adverse lifestyle choices (obesity, lack of exercise, insufficient amount of deep sleep, poor nutrition, excess stress, etc.), as well as possible genetic components (which happen to be **much less causative than environmental factors!).** The remaining chapters of this book delve into what research in these areas has shown, and **what you can do to protect yourself and your family.**

# Cancer in Perspective

*What You Need to Understand
About the Scope of This Book*

———— ★ ★ ★ ————

Every cell in your body is capable of contracting cancer! Therefore, since you have many thousands of types of cells in your body, you have the possibility of contracting one or more of the many thousands of types of cancers! But be aware of the complexities of the tissues of your body: As one example, consider your skin. It is a multi-cell type of tissue, which means that its various layers each are independently comprised of a different cell type, which translates into a susceptibility to a different kind of cancer for the cells of each layer. Furthermore, the tissues and cells of each organ are susceptible to different kinds of cancer, which, collectively, makes for a long list of types of cancers!

As noted in the *Preface,* **from the moment that you were born, your body has been producing more than a million mini cancers every day that are seeking locations in your body to establish toeholds from which to develop into full-blown cancers!** This highlights the **HUGE job** that your immune system has every day – to seek out and kill those mini-cancers! **(Hence, the need to do everything possible to boost the level of functioning of your**

# CANCER

**immune system!)**

It would take many encyclopedia-length volumes to convey all of the known information about cancers, which would be well beyond the scope of this book! The most common cancers in humans are those of the breasts, lungs, mouth/throats, the lymph system, ovaries, prostates, bladders, uteruses and cervixes, skin, and blood cells (white blood cells, red blood cells, etc.).

The focus of this book is to convey information about how to substantially reduce your risks for contracting cancer, and how to improve your odds for surviving cancer if you contract it; however, it is noteworthy that the general principles outlined herein also apply to other well-known, well researched principles:

- How to produce, and then maintain, a sleek, slender **body weight** – within 5 to 10 pounds of your ideal body weight. **Being overweight or obese (that is a Body Mass Index over 30) GREATLY increases your risk not only of cancers, but**

- **also of infections, including the coronavirus COVID-19, as well as your risk of dying from those infections!**

- How to get a sufficient amount of sufficiently demanding **cardio exercise** (that is, endurance exercise in the form of Interval Training) each week,

- How to get a sufficient amount of sufficiently demanding **strength-building exercise** each week,

- How to get a sufficient amount of **deep sleep** virtually every night,

- The importance of getting at least some skin exposure to sunlight each week,

- How to get, and then maintain, **a "can-do"/"will-do" attitude and belief,** including keeping your **stress level(s)** as low as possible,

- How to practice **epigenetic principles** that will activate healthy genes in your genome, and inactivate unhealthy genes in your genome,

- The importance of minimizing (ideally, TOTALLY avoiding) fumes from paints, varnishes, shellacs, etc.), or at least having very robust ventilation when using them, and

- The importance of always practicing **spirituality principles.** (This means that one should treat all living organisms, as well as the environment/ecosystem, with total respect.)

- To add another layer of basic information, realize that there are **three general types of cancer:** basal cell, squamous cell, and malignant melanoma.

- **Basal cell cancer** is the least dangerous kind of cancer. It virtually never spreads (metastasizes) to other tissues and organs. On the very rare occasion that it does metastasize, it is so noteworthy that it is usually reported to a research publication.

- **Squamous cell cancer** is of an intermediate level of

dangerousness.

- By far, **malignant melanoma** is the most dangerous type of cancer. One day, the wife of one of my friends went to her doctor regarding a suspicious growth on one of her calves. Immediately recognizing it as malignant melanoma, her doctor cancelled the rest of his appointments that day, and scheduled emergency surgery for early that afternoon!

Personally, I developed lung cancer a few years ago after almost dying from septic shock following a colonoscopy. Apparently, one or more blood vessels were nicked, which allowed fecal matter to enter into my bloodstream. I survived because, overall, **I had excellent health with respect to cardio exercise, strength-building exercise, nutrition, a positive attitude, and a low level of stress!**

We now (in 2021) have access to published research data which show that imperfect health **GREATLY** increases your risk of infection by COVID-19, and death from it, too! (Note: **These principles are fully relevant to infections and cancers in general** – and this book seeks to show how to minimize these risks and potential impacts on you!)

We wish you well as you work your way through the chapters of this book, and then as you apply their principles to enrich your health and your life in general!

# References

Alegría-Torres, J.A., et al. (June, 2011). Epigenetics and lifestyle.

*Epigenomics, 3*(3), 267-277.

Blair, C.K., et al. (December, 2019). Correlates of poor adherence to a healthy lifestyle among a diverse group of colorectal cancer survivors.

*Cancer Causes & Control, 30*(12), 1327-1339.

Colpani, V., et al. (September, 2018). Lifestyle factors, cardiovascular disease and all-cause mortality in middle aged and elderly women: a systematic review and metanalysis.

*European Journal of Epidemiology, 33*(9), 831-845.

Inaida, S., & Matsuno, S. (April 17, 2020). Previous infection positively correlates to the tumor incidence rate of patients with cancer.

*Cancer Immunology Research, 8*(5),580-586.

Karavasiloglou, N., et al. (June 26, 2019). Healthy lifestyle iinversely associated with mortality in cancer survivors: results from the Third National Health and Nutrition Examination Survey

(NHANES III).

*PLoS One, 14*(6), e0218048 and following.

Lagström, H., et al. (April 1, 2020). Diet quality as a predictor of cardiometabolic disease-free life expectancy: the Whitehall II cohort study.

*American Journal of Clinical Nutrition, 111*(4), 787-794.

Li, Y., et al. (2018). Impact of healthy lifestyle factors on life expectancies in the U.S. population.

*Circulation, 138*(4), 345355 and following.

Li, Y., et al. (January 8, 2020). Healthy lifestyle and life expectancy free of cancer, cardiovascular disease, and type 2 diabetes: prospective cohort study.

*British Medical Journal, 368,* 16669 and following.

Lighter, J., et al., (April 9, 2020). Obesity in patients younger than 60 years is a risk factor for COVID-19 hospital admission.

*Clinical Infectious Diseases,* ciaa415.

Nyberg, S.T., et al. (April 6, 2020). Association of healthy lifestyle with years lived without major chronic diseases.

*JAMA Internal Medicine, 180*(5), 1-10.

Simonnet, A, et al., April 9, 2020. High prevalence of obesity in severe acute respiratory syndrome coronavirus-2 (SARSCOV-2) requiring invasive mechanical ventilation.

*Obesity (Silver Spring).* doi: 10:1002/oby.22831.

Stefan, N., et al. April 23, 2020. Obesity and impaired metabolic health in patients with COVID-19.

*Nature Reviews. Endocrinology,* doi: 10.1038/s41574.

# Chapter Two

# The 8 Foundational Pillars for Best Health

★ ★ ★

In the context of aiming for the healthiest living in order to decrease the odds of contracting a dangerous cancer, it is helpful to focus on practicing **The 8 Foundational Pillars for Best Health:**

### 1. Sleep

For the best, deepest sleep, it is important to utilize one or more background sources for *drowning out unnecessary noise;* you might consider using **fans and/or white noise on your radio** (simply place the tuning dial *between* FM stations on your dial). Also, keep your bedroom as dark as possible by **using heavy, dark drapes,** etc. In addition, **keep the room as cool as possible;** if you or your partner likes it warmer, that person should use an extra blanket. Finally, it is important to institute the practice of **reducing light for at least an hour before "lights out" by turning off <u>all</u> electronic devices** (TVs, cellphones, and all other electronic devices) **for that last hour or so**

**before you plan on going to sleep.** If you generally have night lights on during the night, consider covering their outside with aluminum foil, and/or hiding them around a corner if the layout of your room makes that possible.

2. **Reduce Stress**

If needed, make **a written list of all the sources of stress that you experience – coupled with possible ways of reversing each source of stress.** For example, you could **break a large task into a series of smaller, more manageable tasks,** and then figure out the best way (best order, for example) to put all the pieces together. – Yet another category of stress reduction might require having a heart-to-heart conversation with someone (for example, a boss or an employee) who does not fully understand you, and who does things that raise your stress levels.

3. **Cardio Exercise**

Ideally, **you should have** *three sufficiently demanding cardio workouts each week,* **and virtually never less than two cardio workouts a week, with a day or two of rest between cardio workouts.** You should **do Interval Training,** and choose a machine or activity that you like, and then work up to a level of difficulty (over a period from two weeks to two months – depending on your level of cardio fitness now) such that **you cannot carry on a conversation from the first "sprint" part of the first Interval Cycle – all the way to the end of the cardio workout.** A convenient and effective protocol for each Interval Cycle **is** *30 seconds of all-out sprint,* **followed by** *30 seconds of partial recovery.* Once you are in

# CANCER

great cardio condition, your cardio workout will consist of <u>6 to 8 Interval Cycles</u>, followed by several minutes of cooldown; thus, **your total cardio workout will be no more than about 12 to 13 minutes when you include a minute or two of cool-down at the end, and several minutes of warm-up at the beginning.**

4. <u>**Strength Building Exercise**</u>

In the best of all worlds, you would have **two to three strength-building workouts each week, with at least one day off between workouts. For <u>upper body muscles</u>** (arms, chest, shoulders, upper back muscles), you should **work up to a level such that you do 6 to 10 repetitions (*"reps"*) to the point of muscle failure for each exercise; this means that you are struggling on the last one or two reps and cannot do any more. Once you can do 11 or 12 reps to muscle failure, then it is time to increase the weight or resistance.**

**For your <u>leg exercises</u>,** choose about three exercises for your thighs, such as leg extensions, leg presses, and leg curls. **Choose weights/resistances that allow you to do 15 to 20 reps before reaching the point of muscle failure.**

In addition, you should have at least one exercise or more for each major muscle: for example, the muscles known as biceps, triceps, deltoids (lateral, forward, and rear), trapezius, rhomboids, abdominals, lower back, pectoralis ("pecs"), latissimus dorsi, quadriceps, and hamstrings (also called "thigh biceps").

5. <u>**Nutrition**</u>

A huge amount of misinformation is given to us each day in

magazine articles and books, on blogs and TV programs, etc. This is because nutritionists and other nutrition experts are themselves in total disarray. There are too many "**so-called** *experts*" who are putting out advice that is labelled as "fact," that simply has no support in the scientific literature. And you cannot rely on degrees that these **"experts"** have in the form of alphabet soup after their names; even PhD degrees in nutrition cannot be relied upon, nor can the level of prestige of the PhD-issuing university be relied upon! – "So, where do we go from here?" you might ask.

The answer is that **great nutrition boils down to just a relatively few simple, straight-forward rules.** The most important rule is:

you will have the best health when you

**TRANSFORM**

**YOUR NUTRITION**

**TO 100% PLANT-BASED FOOD!**

& Also

**100% GLUTEN-FREE!**

(Li, 2019; McGrann, 2019)

a.  Fruits:

Eat at least <u>five servings</u> a day. *Serving size* = **½ cup** for fresh fruit, and **¼ cup** for dried fruit.

# CANCER

**b. Vegetables:**

Eat at least <u>five servings</u> a day. *Serving size* = **1 cup** for raw greens, and **½ cup** for cooked greens; for all other vegetables, 1 serving = **½ cup** cooked or raw. Try to incorporate more <u>cruciferous vegetables</u> into your nutrition (kale, broccoli, cabbage, cauliflower, watercress, bok choy). Also, include greens, such as spinach, kale, collard greens, and dandelion greens from your yard if you have not put pesticides on them!

<u>**IMPORTANT NOTE**</u>: **Generally, you will derive more nutrition benefits when you cook these foods, or at least stir fry them for two or so minutes, to breakdown their cellulose cell walls to release key nutrients!**

**c. <u>Nuts & Seeds</u>:**

Eat four or more servings a day and **include at least one serving with each meal to assist with the absorption of oil soluble nutrients.** (I eat 2 or 3 servings of nuts for my brunch, and 3 or 4 servings for my dinner.) For example, lycopene (found in tomatoes, watermelons, etc.) is oily, and is more fully absorbed when consumed with nuts and/or seeds because of the healthy oils in them. *Serving size* = **1 ounce** (a volume that is equivalent to the volume of 18-20 roasted pistachio nuts without their shells). Examples include pumpkin seeds, sunflower seeds, cashews, pistachios, peanuts, and macadamias.

**d. <u>Berries</u>:**

Aim for at least 3 or 4 servings a day, and include at least two varieties. I usually eat blueberries and blackberries. Other varieties include strawberries, raspberries, lingonberries, etc.

e. <u>Variety</u> *is of the utmost importance.*

Be certain to add variety in each of the above groups; this means: one apple, one orange, ½ of a large grapefruit, etc.

<u>Overdoing it on any single food</u>: Just like animals, plants have immune systems. They include poisons for bacteria, viruses, fungi, and parasites. Thus, **if you consume too much of one food, you can experience dangerous side effects.** For example, if you consume too many soybeans in a meal, you can experience dangerous side effects, such as blood clots, etc.! on my "<u>Foods to Avoid List</u> below)," so this should not be an issue for you – though the principle of <u>avoiding consuming large quantities of **ONE FOOD**</u> applies. (Many wrongly assume that eating more of a healthy food means an even healthier result! Never let yourself fall victim to this myth!)

<u>Spiciness</u>: Incorporating very spicy condiments into your daily nutrition may reduce your risk of contracting many cancers by 10% or more! Thus, aim to include spices such as cumin, garlic, hot peppers (cayenne, crushed red peppers, habanero, etc.) in your kitchen concoctions!

<u>Glutens</u>: **Foods made of wheat (including varieties thereof (such as faro, triticale, kamut, and spelt), contain glutens that should be avoided to decrease your risks for multiple sclerosis and celiac disease** if you are predisposed to them (but consult your physician on this), as well as <u>inflammation</u> in general! Furthermore,

realize that **your body may experience negative consequences from glutens, but with NO symptoms**! I strongly recommend that you take the conservative approach and **avoid ALL gluten-containing foods!**

Remember that **glutens are found in food products made from wheat, rye, and barley.**

**SIDE NOTE**: It is impossible to avoid eating GMOs (Genetically Modified Organisms), so do not waste your time trying to avoid them!

Next, be certain to add in **Protein Sources**.

**Protein:** 60 to 70 grams/day. The basic formula for how much you should consume daily: **at least 0.35 grams of protein per pound of body weight; but, also, be certain NOT to consume VERY LARGE QUANTITIES of PROTEIN in a given day!**

*Consider:* **beans in general, lentils, mung beans (also known as moong beans), black-eyed peas, lima beans, nuts, true whole ("unground") grains (such as quinoa, teff, wild rice, and amaranth), but not wheat and varieties thereof, rye, or barley).**

Finally, **TOTALLY** *avoid meat from mammals!* **That is, avoid *all* beef, pork, bison, squirrel, rabbit, lamb, etc.).** On the other hand, an occasional serving of beef, etc. may not hurt your overall health; but see Chapter 24 for more on this, including one reference that challenges this statement!

Bottom Line: **It is much healthier to get all of your protein from** plant sources that are gluten-free!

- a. **Dairy**: <u>Totally avoid</u> **your consumption of dairy products, such as milk, ice cream, animal-based cheeses and yogurts, etc.; these promote cancers!** However, coconut yogurt, for example, is OK.

- b. **Sugars**: **TOTALLY** avoid *ALL* **sugary foods;** they damage every cell in your body, and increase your risks for cancer, type 2 diabetes, dementia, Alzheimer's, and many more diseases. Also, avoid sugar-added foods, such as many dried fruits (exceptions: prunes, apricots, etc.), icing, candy, most fruit juices, pastries, and cold cereals. <u>The Exception</u>: For an hour or so after a demanding workout, some sugary foods, as well as sugar equivalents, will help replenish glycogen stores in your muscles and liver, and do not cause adverse effects. (Richter, E.A., et al. 1985).

- c. **Flour**: **TOTALLY avoid** *ALL* **foods made with flour – both "whole grain" flour and "bleached/white" flour;** these are SUGAR EQUIVALENTS because they are **immediately** converted to sugar in your body via powerful amylase enzymes in your saliva; and their glycemic indices are identical to those of sugars!

  <u>Examples</u>: Breads, pastas, cookies, pretzels, cold cereals, crackers, oatmeal (if you have access to a store that has oat groats, buy the oat groats instead), most "brown rice" (brown rice is OK when it has the same protein and fiber content as wild rice), pastries, cakes, pie crust, etc.

<u>Exceptions</u>: Flours made from almonds and other nuts are OK.

# CANCER

d. **True Whole Grains:** Three or more, servings/day (½ cup cooked true whole grain = 1 serving). **Examples**: Quinoa, teff, amaranth, wild rice, oat groats (**much** healthier than oatmeal!), etc., but totally avoid food made with wheat (and varieties thereof), barley, and rye – which contain glutens.

e. **Egg Yolks:** Eliminate egg yolks because they contain the carcinogenic chemicals choline and lutein. (Tse & Eslick, 2014; Keum, et al., 2015.) Also, see the **Additional Egg Yolk References** at the end of the **REFERENCES** section.

f. **Water and Hydration:**

I once heard a movie star talking with Oprah on TV. The movie star said that she always made sure that she "drank her 9 to 10 glasses of water a day." That movie star had bought into a myth! The truth is that we DO need about 9 to 10 glasses-worth of water a day, but **the water in the foods and drinks that we consume count toward that total consumption amount!**

**The Truth**: Some years ago, two former medical school professors from Dartmouth Medical School were called out of retirement to search the biomedical research literature for data to support the "need for 9 to 10 glasses of water a day" concept. They started with research publications in the early 1900s, and carried through up to their then-current research literature. They found no support for needing to drink 9 to 10 glasses of water a day; however, they did find research data to support the need for about 9 to 10 glasses-worth of water a day <u>when the water came mainly from the foods and drinks</u>

<u>that a person consumed</u>.

I recommend that all of us eat at least 5 servings of fruit, at least 5 servings of vegetables, and at least 3 servings of berries each day. This, when combined with one or two glasses or cups of liquid a day will provide a sufficient amount of water each day.

g. **<u>Alcohol Consumption</u>**:

**<u>TOTALLY avoid *ALL* alcoholic drinks</u>!** Your liver converts alcohol to acetaldehyde, a potent carcinogen. We used to think that *some* alcohol was okay, even beneficial, in decreasing the risks for developing clots, strokes, heart attacks, etc.; however, the latest research shows that the supposed benefits are minimal at best, and that the risk of getting cancer from consuming alcohol is strong!

h. **What About <u>Canned Foods</u>?**

**<u>TOTALLY avoid *ALL* canned food</u> (that is foods in <u>metal containers</u>) because their plastic linings contain the highly carcinogenic BPA (bis-phenol A), and/or other dangerous chemical plasticizers that are also carcinogenic, and that cause miscarriages in pregnant women!**

i. **Other Dietary Considerations**

**<u>Rules for diabetics</u>:** For those of you who are prediabetic, or genetically prone to type 2 diabetes, eat fresh or frozen fruits and root vegetables (carrots, turnips, rutabagas, etc.) **only** as <u>part of an overall healthy meal</u>. Also, TOTALLY avoid ALL sugary foods and all foods made of flour! (See comments in

# CANCER

above sections.)

j. **Multi-Vitamins & Supplements:** Many studies show that people who take multi-vitamins and other supplements are no healthier than those who take none! Furthermore, some studies show increased risks for some types of cancer! (Watson, 2011). [Note: James Watson, was the Nobel Laureate for being the co-discoverer of the alpha-helical structure of DNA. His 2011 article points out research results that show that taking "anti-oxidant" supplements is detrimental to your health!]

k. **Some exceptions**

**Vitamin D3** [no more than about 800 to 1,000 International units (IU) a day], and **Vitamin B12** (no more than about 6 or 8 micrograms a day in pill form) are exceptions to the above generalizations.

**Iron** is an exception for pregnant women.

## Notes:

1. Use the serving size information in the Nutrition Sections above only as **a *general* guideline for adults;** that is, there is <u>no</u> *reason* to measure out *precise volumes* or weights every time you eat!

2. It is important that you recognize that **great nutrition also has positive effects on both your <u>mood</u> and your <u>mental health</u>!** (Lin & Su, 2007; Lasalle, et al., 2018; Bloch & Hannestad, 2012;

Masuoka, et al., 2017; Lin, et al., 2012; Kaplan, et al., 2007; Vecchioli, et al., 2018; Amen, et al., 2013; Colin, et al., 2003).

## Creating Your Shopping List

Before you go grocery shopping, **prepare a <u>detailed list</u> of healthy foods that you will buy, and <u>*stick to your list*</u> because <u>you and the others in your household will eat *whatever* you have on the shelves</u>!** It is the result of the normal functioning of a primitive part of your brain! In other words, do not fight this tendency; rather, compensate for it by **sticking to your shopping list!**

## Eating 5 or 6 Small Meals a Day

Many nutritionists and dietitians recommend eating five or six small meals (instead of the traditional 3 meals a day) because each meal that is digested supposedly produces a small burst of increased calorie burn. However, recent (and better designed) studies show that this effect is minimal or non-existent. I only have two meals a day: a huge brunch, and dinner – which saves me a nice chunk of time that I can utilize for other things.

## Losing Excess Weight

**If you want to lose excess weight, be sure to develop a vigorous <u>*Interval Training* program</u>, combined with a great <u>strength-building program</u>.** Your resulting increased <u>after-burn calories</u>

will reward you with a healthier body, and *much* **shorter cardio workouts,** especially if you avoid swimming and cool or cold showers afterwards (which would decrease or eliminate the otherwise beneficial after-burn calories that reflect an increased internal body temperature and increased Basal Metabolic Rate (BMR))!

## Cutting and Washing Food

Be sure to **thoroughly <u>wash the *outer parts* of any food that you are about to eat</u>.** For example, wash the grapefruit that you are about to cut in half and eat. Have you ever watched the food merchandizer polish the apples, grapefruits, oranges, cucumbers, etc. before positioning them on the shelves? The polishing with the wax on a cloth just spreads germs to each piece of food that he/she treats!

## Raw vs. Cooked

Many books and articles have been written that advertise the supposed health benefits of eating **raw foods.** What a **huge mistake of** *facts!* The cells of plants are made of cellulose, which, in effect, traps nutrients inside those cells; thus, if incomplete chewing occurs (which is the result virtually all the time for all of us!), then **cooking (steaming is OK, too) is required to tear down those cellulose walls, which means that more internal nutrients will be beneficially released into your body** when you consume the food (applicable to vegetables, but not fruits)!

An excellent review article (that cited 88 references) concluded that *some* vegetables are more healthful when eaten cooked, and *other* vegetables are more healthful when eaten raw. In addition, nutrition benefits can also vary, for example, depending on how they are prepared. Thus, a simple conclusion on which is more healthy – raw versus cooked – is not possible! (Link & Potter, 2004.)

You may be wondering what all the fuss is about Sugar and Sugar Equivalents in the Nutrition sections above. Allow me to make the following comments.

1. High levels of sugar (glucose) can damage cells in *any* part of your body.

2. High blood sugar levels can potentially push your body over the line – to make you a type 2 diabetic.

3. Even if your body does *not* transform into full-blown type 2 diabetes from consuming sugary and flour-based foods, *any* of the organs and tissues of your body still potentially can be injured with diabetic-type damage and with no outwardly noticeable effects!

4. Diabetic-type damage (even for the *non-diabetic*) can include, for example, one or more of:

    - **peripheral neuropathy** (including **gangrene,** which would require emergency (life-threatening) amputation of the affected tissue in the limb or other body part)
    - **loss of hearing** (or diminution of your hearing)

# CANCER

- **loss of eyesight** (or diminution of your sight)

- <u>hair loss</u> virtually always (except for special medical situations) **is a sign of <u>diabetic-type damage to the hair follicles</u> that have stopped producing normal, mature hair;** thus, whether you are a female or a male, and the hair growing from your scalp is largely missing (that is, not dense like it was when you were young), then **you most likely are an un-diagnosed diabetic, a prediabetic, or at least a potential diabetic.** – So, **virtually all <u>bald men</u> whom you see everywhere got that way from poor nutrition, specifically from too much sugar and sugar equivalents (i.e., sugar- and flour-based foods, etc.).**

- <u>PCOS</u> ("Polycystic Ovary Syndrome") is a condition in which a woman loses hair, and usually also has some amount of male-like facial hair – possibly including a beard and a mustache

- **loss of taste** (or diminution of your sense of taste)

- **sexual dysfunction** (this can occur for either gender)

- **itching** (medical term: pruritus)

- greatly **increased risk for dementia and Alzheimer's Disease**

- **greatly increased risk for <u>developing cancers in general</u>!**

5. The last point (about the risk for cancers) is of particular interest for the focus of this book. In some studies, **incredible**

results (*reversal*, as well as *conversion of cancer cells to normal cells*) **have been achieved by nutrition alone** by what I call **"sugar starving" the cancer cells**! (Han, et al., 2016; Meyerhardt, et al., 2012; Rock, et al., 2012; Merganthaler, et al., 2012; Ballard-Barbash, et al., 2012; Onodera, et al., 2014; Graham, et al., 2012; Wiegl, et al., 2018; Lin, et al., 2015; Fridlender, et al., 2015). (See also Chapters 4, 8, and 14.)

As noted earlier, nutrition is especially important not only for your general overall health, but also for reducing your risk for cancers, as well as your odds of reversing cancer if you develop it. Having said this, we can make **a few additional critical predictions and prescriptions**, which, when followed, will *further decrease your risk of getting cancer, and also increase your success for reversing cancer if you have it or if you develop it.*

**To the extent that your immune system protects your body from cancers, even better cancer-fighting abilities will result from adding other strategies that will boost your immune system's function.** This is the basis for **all** of the chapters of this book. Thus, **exercise, sleep, avoiding gasoline and exhaust fumes, etc. are covered so that you can further increase your odds of success in preventing and/or reversing cancer.**

Although it was mentioned earlier in this chapter, it is worth reemphasizing that **you and everyone else on the planet have had millions of cancers and cancer-causing viruses, etc. in your body every day from the moment that you were born!** And your immune system destroys these millions of cancers every day! Thus, adopting a healthy lifestyle will boost the level of function of your immune system! [See Chapter 27 for a discussion of the scientific data on this in the relatively new field of **Epigenetics**.] Great nutrition is also critical for the best mental health, as is shown in a review that concludes that **the best nutrition greatly increases the odds of happiness for humans** (Lassalle, et al., 2018).

## Things to Avoid!

Vitamin A, beta-carotene, vitamin E, selenium, iron (except for pregnant women), corn and corn-containing foods, egg yolks, and copper; keep salt utilization to a minimum.

## Giving Back

When you help others in need (defined as those who are less well-off than you), you are applying spirituality principles that will make you a better, more compassionate, more fully understanding person. In fact, you might well find that you gain more benefit than those whom you help!

You need not necessarily spend oodles of time. For example, you might regularly help a neighborhood kid with his homework, or grocery shop for a frail, elderly neighbor.

## Attitude

**Attitude is all-important because it reveals who you *really* are! If you have a great attitude, you will always treat others with respect, kindness, and goodwill.** Attitude can also reveal if you have the right motives on various aspects of life – for example, having the discipline to study hard while a student in college, to work for a job promotion, or to start your own business – to cite just a few examples!

## Spirituality

**Spirituality is all about respect for life – that is, ALL life, including people, the animals around us, ecosystems, and, ultimately, the entire planet!** For example, **the spiritually motivated person will not litter, will not be quick to anger, and will always treat others with appreciation and respect.** The spiritually motivated person will work to move things forward – and *not* stand in the way of progress and enlightenment!

Consult other references below that relate to nutrition, exercise, and other cancer risks (Ford, et al., 2016; O'Keefe, et al., 2015; Koeth, et al., 2013; Boeing, et al., 2013; Vivante, et al., 2012; Key, 2011; Solfrizzi, et al., 2011; Sluijs, et al., 2010; Uribarri, et al., 2010; Sinha, et al., 2009; Peppa & Raptis, 2008; Key & Spencer, 2007; Zheng, et al., 2015; Johannson, et al., 2018; Lu, et al., 2016; Thomson, et al., 2014; Mourouti, et al., 2017; Michaëlsson, K., et al., 2017; Michaëlsson, K., et al., 2014).

Now, you are ready to move on to the next chapters!

# References

Amen, D.G., et al. (2013). Effects of brain-directed nutrients on cerebral blood flow and neuropsychological testing: A randomized, double-blind, placebo-controlled, crossover trial.

*Advances in Mind-Body Medicine, 27*(2), 24-33.

Ballard-Barbash, R., et al. 2012. Physical activity, biomarkers, and disease outcomes in cancer survivors: A systematic review.

*Journal of the National Cancer Institute, 104*(11), 815-840.

Barbour, K.A., et al. (2007). Exercise as a treatment for depression and other psychiatric disorders: A review.

*Journal of Cardiopulmonary Rehabilitation and Prevention, 27*(6), 359-367.

Bloch. M.H., & Hannestad, J. (2012). Omega-3 fatty acids for the treatment of depression: Systematic review and meta-analysis.

*Molecular Psychiatry, 17*(12), 1272-1282.

Boeing, H., et al. (2012). Critical review: Vegetables and fruit in the prevention of chronic diseases.

*European Journal of Nutrition, 51*(6), 637-663.

[Note: This excellent review contains 298 references.]

Colin, A., et al. (2003). Lipids, depression, and suicide.

*Encephale, 29*(1), 49-58. (Article in French).

Ford, C.T., et al. (2016). Identification of (poly)phenol treatments that modulate the release of pro-inflammatory cytokines by human lymphocytes.

*The British Journal of Nutrition, 115*(10), 1699-1710.

Fridlender, M., et al. (2015). Plant derived substances with anticancer activity: From folklore to practice.

*Frontiers in Plant Science, 6,* 799 and following.

Gradari, S., et al. (2016). Can exercise make you smarter, happier, and have more neurons? A Hormetic perspective.

*Frontiers in Neuroscience, 10,* 93 and following.

Graham, N.A., et al. (2012). Glucose deprivation activates a metabolic and signaling amplification loop leading to cell death.

*Molecular Systems Biology, 8,* 589 and following.

Han, J., et al. (2016). Interleukin-6 stimulates aerobic glycolysis by regulating PFKFB3 at early stage of colorectal cancer.

*International Journal of Oncology, 48*(1), 215-224.

Li, William W. (2019). Eat to Beat Disease: The New Science of How Your Body Can Heal Itself. [Book]

# CANCER

Johannson, I., et al. (2018). Dairy intake revisited – associations between dairy intake and lifestyle related cardiometabolic risk factors in a high milk consuming population.

*Nutrition Journal, 17*(1), 110 and following.

Kaplan, B.J., et al. (2007). Vitamins, minerals, and mood.

*Psychological Bulletin, 133*(5), 747-760.

Keum, N., et al. (2015). Egg intake and cancers of the breast, ovary and prostate: A dose-response meta-analysis of prospective observational studies.

*The British Journal of Nutrition, 114*(7), 1099-1107.

Key, T.J. (2011). Fruit and vegetables and cancer risk.

*British Journal of Cancer, 104*(1), 6-11.

Key, T.J., & Spencer, E.A. (2007). Carbohydrates and cancer: An overview of the epidemiological evidence.

*European Journal of Clinical Nutrition, 61*(Suppl 1), S112-S121.

Koeth, R.A., et al. (2013). Intestinal microbiota metabolism of *L*-carnitine, a nutrient in red meat, promotes atherosclerosis.

*Nature Medicine, 19*(5), 576-585.

Lassale, C., et al. (2018). Healthy dietary indices and risk of depressive outcomes: A systematic review and meta-analysis of observational studies. *Molecular Psychiatry, 24*, 965-986.

**[This review concludes that those with the best nutrition are**

**happier and have better mental health.]**

Li, William W. (2019. *Eat to Beat Disease: The New Science of How Your Body Can Heal Itself.*

Lin, P.H., et al. (2015). Nutrition, dietary interventions and prostate cancer: The latest evidence.

*BMC Medicine, 13,* 3 and following.

**[From this review of 197 references, these authors conclude that a healthy dietary pattern consists of consuming lots of fruits and vegetables, and consuming extremely limited quantities of refined carbohydrates, total fat, saturated fats, and cooked red meats (that is, meat from mammals).]**

Lin, P-Y., & Su, K-P. (2007). A meta-analytic review of double-blind, placebo-controlled trials of antidepressant efficacy of omega-3 fatty acids.

*Journal of Clinical Psychiatry, 68*(7), 1056-1061.

Lin, P-Y., et al. (2012). Are omega-3 fatty acids anti-depressants or just mood-improving agents?

*Molecular Psychiatry, 17*(12), 1161-1163.

Link, L.B., & Potter, J.D. (2004). Raw versus cooked vegetables and cancer risk.

*Cancer Epidemiology, Biomarkers & Prevention, 13*(9), 1422-1435.

Lu, W., et al. (2016). Dairy products intake and cancer mortality risk: A meta-analysis of 11 population-based cohort studies.

*Nutrition Journal, 15*(1): 91 and following.

Masuoka, Y.J., et al. (2017). Dietary fish, n-3 polyunsaturated fatty acid consumption, and depression in Japan: A population based prospective cohort study.

*Translational Psychiatry, 7*(9), e1242 and following.

McGrath, Debbie. (2019). *The Accidental Cure. The SECRET Treatment your doctor will not tell you. The true story of my recovery from Multiple Sclerosis and Celiac Disease.* Imagination Press, Columbia, Maryland.

Mergenthaler, P., et al. (2012). Mitochondrial hexokinase II (HKII) and phosphoprotein enriched astrocytes (PEA15) form a molecular switch governing cellular fate depending on the metabolic state.

*Proceedings of the National Academy of Sciences, 109*(5), 1518-1523.

Meyerhardt, J.A., et al. (2012). Glycemic load and cancer recurrence and survival in patients with stage III colon cancer:

Findings from CALGB 89803.

*Journal of the National Cancer Institute, 104*(22), 1702-1711.

Richter, E.A., et al. (1985). Increased glucose uptake after exercise. No need for insulin during exercise.

*Diabetes, 34*(10), 1041-1048.

# Additional Egg Yolk References

---   ★ ★ ★   ---

Dehghan, M., et al. (2020). Association of egg intake with blood lipids, cardiovascular disease, and mortality in 177,000 people in 50 countries.

*American Journal of Clinical Nutrition, 111*(4), 795-803.

DiBella, M., et al, (2020). Choline intake as supplement or as a component of eggs increases plasma choline and reduces interleukin-6 without modifying plasma cholesterol in participants with metabolic syndrome.

*Nutrients, 12*(10), 3120 and following.

Djoussé, L., et al. (2020). Egg consumption and risk of coronary artery disease in the Million Veteran Program.

*Clinical Nutrition, 39*(9), 2842-2847.

Drouin-Chartier, J.P., et al. (2020). Egg consumption and type 2 diabetes: Findings from 3 large US cohort studies of men and women and a systematic review and meta-analysis of prospective cohort studies.

*American Journal of Clinical Nutrition, 112*(3), 619-630.

Hills, Jr., R.D., et al. (2019). Gut microbiome: Profound implications for diet and disease.

*Nutrients, 11*(7), 1613 and following.

MacDonald, C.J., et al. (2020). Cholesterol and egg intakes, and risk of hypertension in a large prospective cohort of French women.

*Nutrients, 12*(5), 1350 and following.

Maki, K.C., et al. (2020). Effects of substituting eggs for high-carbohydrate breakfast foods on the cardiometabolic risk-factor profile in adults at risk for type 2 diabetes mellitus.

*European Journal of Clinical Nutrition, 74*(5), 784-795.

Tang, H., et al. (2020). Egg consumption and stroke risk: A systematic review and dose-response meta-analysis of prospective studies.

*Frontiers in Nutrition, 7,* 153 and following.

Tong, T.Y.N., et al. (2020). The associations of major foods and fibre with risks of ischaemic and haemorragic stroke: A prospective study of 418,329 participants in the EPIC cohort across nine European countries.

*European Heart Journal, 41*(28), 2632-2640.

Zhong, V.W., et al. (2020). Associations of processed meat, unprocessed red meat, poultry, or fish intake with incident cardiovascular disease and all-cause mortality.

*JAMA Internal Medicine, 180*(4), 503-512.

# Chapter Three

# Additional Foundations of Good Health

★ ★ ★

This book features **13 components, <u>ALL</u> of which must be implemented meticulously in order to provide you with the best odds for preventing and reversing cancer!** the Ultimate Cancer Prevention and Cancer Reversal Program of Chapter 1 covered **The 8 Foundational Pillars for Best Health.** Five components remain. Of particular interest, note that Chapter 16 discusses the "Weakest Link" concept as it applies to your health – explaining why even **<u>just one</u> weak link** in your health practices can set you up for poor overall health!

The reference cited below provides an example of a study in which **diet and lifestyle factors affect cancer progression and the risk of dying.** This is an excellent reference with which to dive into the cancer literature.

As mentioned above, this Ultimate Cancer Prevention and

# CANCER

Cancer Reversal Program focuses on **showing YOU how you can fit into your super busy schedule _the healthy, BARE MINIMUM_ in each of a variety of critical categories.** Once you establish a _life-healthy_ weekly schedule, and master these components (actually, mainly 3 components remain because Weight Loss, as you will discover in Chapter 5, will already have been taken care of and realized when you followed the prescriptions laid out in Chapters 4, 6, 7, and 8 of this book), creating your weekly schedule will be much easier!

I strongly suggest that you consult your doctor before making the changes outlined in this book. Your question to her/him should be along the lines of:

**"Is there any compelling reason why I should not undertake a program of <u>gradually</u> increasing the level of my exercise, and <u>gradually</u> changing my nutrition to a super healthy nutrition program?"**

The reason this is important is that you could have a medical condition for which exercise is contraindicated (a relatively rare occurrence), or for which such nutritional changes should be monitored closely, and/or with certain guidelines because of medications that you may be taking.

# Reference

Peisch, S.F., et al. (2017). Prostate cancer progression and mortality: A review of diet and lifestyle factors.

*World Journal of Urology, 35*(6), 867-874.

# Chapter Four

## Various Definitions of "GRADUALLY" and Some Specifics About Making Health Transitions

---  ★ ★ ★  ---

Not only will the definition of "gradually" vary according to area, but also vary according to where you and your health currently stand at the beginning of your health transformation. It is important to start out gradually when you are making healthy changes in your lifestyle. This chapter focuses on how to do this successfully. Do not beat yourself up if and when you have lapses; just change your mindset (Chapter 10), and remember all of the reasons "why" you want to lead a healthy existence. This change in your lifestyle is for you, your family, your friends, etc. Following the plan below will help you gage your performance. However, as with any exercise plan, first consult with your physician.

# DOC WILSON, PhD

## For <u>NUTRITION</u>

| <u>Type of Person</u> | <u>Weeks to Transition</u> |
|---|---|
| **most people:** | 2 weeks to transition to healthy nutrition |
| **a minority of people:** | 3 to 4 weeks to transition to healthy nutrition |

## For CARDIO EXERCISE (Interval Training)

| | |
|---|---|
| the sedentary person: | 8 to 12 weeks |
| the sporadic exerciser: | 5 to 6 weeks |
| consistent, low-level exerciser: | 4 to 6 weeks |
| consistent, high-level exerciser: | ~ 2 weeks, or less |

## For STRENGTH-BUILDING EXERCISE

| | |
|---|---|
| the sedentary person: | 6 to 8 weeks |
| the sporadic exerciser: | 4 to 5 weeks |
| consistent, low-level exerciser: | 3 to 4 weeks |
| consistent, high-level exerciser: | 2 weeks, or less |

# Chapter Five

# The Biochemistry of Cancer, and Why Sugar and "Sugar Equivalents" (including "Undeclared Sugars") are So Dangerous to Your Health

---  ★ ★ ★ ---

Cancer cells differ from normal cells in several ways. **First, cancer cells have a higher metabolic rate than normal cells** (Rhee, et al., 2019).

**Second, cancer cells have defective, non-functioning mitochondria, which cannot release energy stored in the normal food break-down products via the usual Krebs Cycle** (also called the *Tricarboxylic Acid Cycle,* or the *TCA Cycle*). The Krebs cycle is the sequence of reactions by which most living cells generate energy during the process of aerobic respiration. In normal cells, mitochondria are referred to as the "power houses" of the cell.

**Third, because their mitochondria are useless, cancer cells must rely on *glycolysis,* which breaks down glucose (which comes into the cancer cells from the blood; glucose in the blood is also known as *blood sugar*) to release energy. The biochemical end products that result after releasing energy are water and carbon dioxide. *Glycolysis* occurs inside the cells, but outside of the mitochondria.

High blood levels of glucose will fuel glycolysis in cancer cells, but the high glucose levels will also cause glucose molecules to stick to cell membranes throughout a person's body. The *stuck* glucose molecules (*stuck* covalently by chemical bonds) then are converted, by a series of enzymatic reactions, to the sugar alcohol known as *sorbitol.*

The "-ol" in sorbitol refers to the alcohol group -OH (also known as a hydroxyl group). Hydroxyl groups have a hydrogen molecule attached covalently to an oxygen molecule. Cell membranes have inside and outside portions that are electrically charged, and that attract water molecules (and are thus *hydrophilic* – loving water). **The hydroxyl group on sorbitol is soluble *both* in water and in oil,** which defines the physical character of the *interior* of a cell membrane. Because of this dual functionality of the hydroxyl group on sorbitol, **if sorbitol is in high amounts on a cell's membrane, it will pierce the cell membrane, and cause *leakage* of the cell's interior fluid out into the surrounding extracellular fluid.**

Inside a normal cell, the fluid is high in potassium, and low in sodium. On the other hand, the extracellular fluid is just the opposite: high in sodium and low in potassium. (The differences are referred to as *ion gradients*.) One effect of the differences between the respective ion concentrations <u>inside</u> of the cell, compared to the concentrations of those ions <u>outside</u> of the cell, is **a** *membrane potential* **of about 100 millivolts negative on the inside of the cell.** When leakage destroys the sodium and the potassium gradients, **the membrane potential is also destroyed, which contributes to <u>the death</u>** of what previously had been a healthy cell.

This means that the net effect of sorbitol is to kill cells in the body of the host. What is critical is to realize that **every cell in a person's body** is potentially susceptible to death by sorbitol, but in a given person, some tissues may become susceptible before other tissues and cells. However, **in a diabetic, often one of the first symptoms is** *<u>peripheral neuropathy</u>* **– which refers to nerve damage in the extremities: usually the feet first. If not treated soon enough, dangerous, life-threatening gangrene can set in – requiring immediate amputation of the affected area(s).**

This example emphasizes the importance of healthy living. It is worth noting that **type 2 diabetes is not only preventable,** *but also reversible* **if it is addressed early – that is, before any permanent damage has occurred.** Therefore, it is critical to avoid sugary foods, as well as foods made of *sugar equivalents* (food made of flour of any kind). Such foods should be on **your** *junk food list.*

Foods that should be on **your** *<u>junk food list</u>* include **all pastas, cookies, cold cereals, cakes, pie dough, most pie fillings, pretzels, breads, pastries, and all other flour-based foods.** Other foods that should also be on **your** *junk food list* include **all soft drinks** (both sugared and artificially sugared), **all deep-fried foods** (think French fries, fried chicken, etc.), any foods that contain artificial sweeteners, and **juices** (which almost always have **added sugar**). Generally, for the average non-diabetic person, eating whole, fresh fruits does not cause huge, dangerous up-ticks in blood glucose; however, **a diabetic should eat fruit and root veggies (turnips, rutabagas, etc.) only as <u>part of an overall healthy meal</u> to minimize any up-ticks in their blood glucose levels.** Also, the nutritious part of potatoes is the skin; the pulpy interior is starch that is a sugar equivalent.

**Special Note:** Recent studies have found that **<u>eating nuts with a meal will prevent or greatly reduce high rises in blood glucose</u>**. – Yet another great reason to include nuts in every meal! (Moreira, et al., 2014; Del Gabb, et al., 2015; Yu, et al., 2016; Luu, et al., 2015; Weng, et al., 2016.)

Another powerful weapon to prevent and/or reverse type 2 diabetes is **High Intensity Interval Training** that is mentioned above in Chapter 1.

Be sure to **consult your physician** *before* **making any of these changes, and <u>work up *gradually* for the Interval Training</u>.** In addition, **your body will also benefit from including a good strength-building exercise program.** That is, **an exercise program that incorporates both strength-building and cardio exercise provides the greatest health benefits!**

# References

Del Gabb, L.C., et al. (2015). Effect of tree nuts on blood lipids, apolipoproteins, and blood pressure: Systematic review, metanalysis, and dose response of 61 controlled intervention studies.

*American Journal of Clinical Nutrition, 102(6), 1347-1356.*

Luu, H.N., et al. (2015). Prospective evaluation of nut/peanut consumption with total and cause-specific mortality.

*JAMA Internal Medicine, 175(5), 86-96.*

Moreira Alves, R.D., et al. (2014). High-oleic peanuts: New perspective to attenuate glucose homeostasis disruption and inflammation related to obesity.

*Obesity (Silver Spring, MD), 22(9), 1981-1988.*

Rhee, H., et al. (2019). Metabolic syndrome and prostate cancer: A review of complex interplay amongst various endocrine factors in the pathophysiology and progression of prostate cancer.

*Hormones & Cancer, 7(2), 75-83.*

Weng, Y.Q., et al. (2016). Association between nut consumption and coronary heart disease.

*Coronary Artery Disease, 27*(3), 227-232.

Yu, Z., et al. (2016). Association between nut consumption and inflammatory biomarkers.

*American Journal of Clinical Nutrition, 104*(3), 722-728.

# Chapter Six

# Body Weight and Weight Loss

---- ★★★ ----

Perhaps you have been a regular member of a gym for 4 or 5 years or longer, and have seen on the cardio exercise machines (usually a variety of elliptical machines, bicycles, and treadmills) individuals whose body weight has remained unchanged over time, or, worse, has increased. Maybe you viewed such human examples as persons *"doing what was necessary and appropriate, but getting ineffective results,"* **which could have made you feel disheartened because, you, too, seemed to be fighting a losing battle with** *your* **weight!**

In this chapter you will learn why so many people *miss the mark* when it comes to losing excess weight!

For starters, gym personnel (including Personal Trainers) almost always have **not** been trained in the area of weight loss, or, if they have been so trained, they have not been trained with scientific research-supported knowledge about all aspects of exercise science. They may have five or six (or more) certifications from the more than 15 certifying entities, and incorrectly believe that they now are *trained professionals* who are knowledgeable. In addition, some have been sucked into believing many of the myths that are told or spread in books, in magazines, and on television and the Internet; many have also been blinded by best-selling authors who have made millions of dollars by pawning off inaccurate information to you, the consumer! In my experience, **the only *regular* area of exercise that usually *has all its ducks in a row* is cycling classes,** in which **Interval Training** is often practiced. In addition, *some* aerobic dance classes have somewhat effective, to very effective, weight loss programs.

From the title of this chapter and the reference to Interval Training in the previous paragraph, I am sure that you know that <u>*Interval Training is at least one of the critical keys to weight loss success!*</u> – So, let us get started so that you not only learn the key elements of an effective Interval Training exercise program, but also *why* each of those elements is so important!

**First,** let us review a few definitions.

**Interval Training** – Cardio exercise in which the exerciser alternates between

- **more difficult work** (that is, faster, bigger resistance, and/or greater slope/incline)

and

- **lesser work** (that is, a period of recovery or partial recovery).

**Interval Cycle** – one stretch of more difficult work, followed by a stretch of recovery or partial recovery.

**Second, 3 basic questions you may be asking:**

*How many Interval Cycles* should you have in your cardio routine?

What *level of difficulty* should you have in your cardio routine?

What machine or activity should you use for your cardio routine?

The *number* of Interval Cycles that you do might only be one or two if you are not already in fairly good cardio condition, and up to six to eight if you are in good or great cardio condition. Similarly, the *level of difficulty* should be in line with the level of your cardio conditioning.

**The machines *and/or* activities should be whatever you like:** taking vigorous aerobic dance or cycling classes, using an elliptical machine, running on a treadmill, running on a hard surface (such as asphalt or concrete), running on a soft surface (such as grass), running on the level, sprinting up hills, and so forth. However, you should **also consider <u>the effect of your selected cardio routine(s) on your various joints</u>** (hips, knees, vertebras and inter-vertebral disks, feet, etc.), and **select more "joint-gentle" exercises** that are still highly effective for cardio training, but that are less likely to harm your joints long-term.

**If you have *any* joint issues or other potential medical issues in these body areas, use elliptical machines or bicycles (either**

stationary bikes or road bikes) for your cardio workouts.** If you really love running outdoors, try to find places (trails, etc.) that have **soft surfaces** (grass, sand, soil, etc.). In addition, **you can reduce joint impact by running _up_ hills, or running on a treadmill** _with the incline ramped up_.

As you get in better and better condition, simply increase the level of difficulty and the number of Interval Cycles that you do. **Once you reach a relatively high level of cardio fitness, you will need to be doing only six to eight Interval Cycles in a given workout.** This generally means that **you will be doing no more than 10 minutes of cardio exercise** (and _never_ more than 14 or 15 minutes _including_ your warm-up and cool-down segments!) You can take three to five minutes to warm-up your body's muscles before starting your Interval Training workout if you wish. The math (assuming 30 seconds fast/hard, and 30 seconds of partial recovery):

**6 Interval Cycles:**

1 minute each, plus 2 minutes of cool-down = **8 minutes**

**8 Interval Cycles:**

1 minute each, plus 2 minutes of cool-down = **10 minutes**

**10 Interval Cycles:**

1 minute each, plus 2 minutes of cool-down = **12 minutes**

**Third, how often should you do your Interval Training?**

Answer: Somewhere from every other day (for example, Monday, Wednesday, Friday, Sunday, Tuesday, etc.) to every third day (for example, Monday, Thursday, Sunday, Wednesday, etc.). In between these two options is three days a week on an every-other-day basis (for example, Monday, Wednesday, Friday; or Monday, Wednesday, Saturday; or Tuesday, Thursday, Sunday; etc.).

**Why is Interval Training the Very Best Cardio Exercise for Losing Excess Weight?** The reason is that **it produces** *a lot* of **afterburn calories**! When you exercise at an intense level (as, ultimately, you will do when you reach the height of your Interval Training program), your body temperature will rise, which is saying the same thing as **increasing your Basal Metabolic Rate (BMR), and increasing the number of calories that your body burns.** With a great Interval Training workout, <u>**your BMR may be elevated for 15 hours or more**</u> after ending your workout – as long as *you do <u>not</u> go swimming* and *do <u>not</u> take a cool or cold shower afterwards!* If you need to shower, take as warm a shower as you can get away with (socially speaking)! You obviously *do not want to smell like a horse for a business meeting* that was scheduled immediately after your workout!

## Some important <u>Notes</u> concerning Interval Training

<u>Note 1:</u> Ideally, for best results, you should be **driving your heart rate as high as possible and getting out of breath to the extent that you cannot carry on a conversation!** However, our Federal Government still has on the books the recommendation that exercisers should be able to carry on a conversation while exercising!

Do not be fooled by this huge myth!

**Note 2: Do not rely on any of the more than half a dozen formulas for "maximum heart rate as a function of age!"** If you were to limit your heart rate to any of the values predicted by these various formulas (as many cardio machines make available), **your heart would actually be getting weaker and weaker with each passing year!** Once you are doing very demanding workouts, your maximum heart rate achieved while doing your Interval Training cardio workout should exceed *all* of the heart rate values predicted by these formulas! **Just *go as hard as you can* for the difficult part (*the sprint portion*) of each Interval Cycle!**

**[Sub-Note 2A: Your maximum heart rate is determined by the strength of your leg muscles,** which *push your venous blood toward your heart;* your heart then increases its rate of beating to accommodate the in-coming blood. This is known as the Bainbridge reflex.]

**Note 3:** Some people think that a high degree of **sweating** during a cardio workout is evidence of doing a sufficiently demanding cardio workout. Do not let yourself be deceived by this fallacy; rather, rely on **the highest heart rate that you can muster, and heavy breathing!**

**Note 4:** See Chapter 7 (next) for **the optimum order** for doing the exercises in your exercise routine.

**Note 5:** If you live or work in a rather confined space and spend a large portion of your day being relatively sedentary, be sure to **get**

up and move about for 5 or 10 minutes, ideally, every 45 to 60 minutes. This practice will not only decrease your risk for dangerous – even life-threatening – DVTs (**Deep Vein Thromboses,** which are *blood clots!*), but will also help your body **burn an extra 300 or more calories per day** just from moving about in this manner. You should also generalize this principle to sitting on long airplane flights, etc.!

**Note 6**: Many cardio machines have **built-in cardio programs** that you can engage with the mere push of a button. I recommend that you disregard these programs, and, instead, *select the manual option.*

The problem with the built-in cardio programs is that they are based on inaccurate heart rate formulas! If you were to use them, your heart rate would not reach the high levels required for optimum results! In particular, the so-called **"Fat Burning" heart rate zone** absurdly *under*estimates where your heart rate needs to be!!!

**Note 7**: I recommend **using your own heart rate monitor for your cardio exercise.** One brand that has served my clients well (and me, too) is Polar™. For women, Polar™ also sells a bra with cutouts for the chest strap (that has the sensor for the heart rate); this serves to prevent the chest strap from sliding too far down the torso. The most important parameters to track (but *only* if you like doing this sort of thing!) are, for a given interval, **your *highest heart rate*** (which occurs 5 to 20 seconds after reaching your peak speed), and **your *coupled peak speed.*** As you progressively get in better cardio condition, **your peak heart rate will drop for the same or greater**

level of difficulty (resistance, incline, etc.), which <u>proves that your heart is getting stronger</u> – often from one workout to the next! This is an absolutely GREAT way to experience and quantitatively appreciate the fruits of your exercise program!

<u>Note 8</u>: Your body weight is critical to your health. If you have excess exterior fat, then you also have excess fat inside your abdomen (intra-abdominal fat – also called **omentum fat** or **visceral fat**). With excess weight, you almost certainly have a **fatty liver,** and this interferes with your liver's ability to function normally; it also **increases your odds of developing type 2 diabetes, cancers,** and many other maladies – in part because the excess fat prevents your liver from pulling sugar out of your blood.

In addition, **with excess omentum fat, your pancreas will not function properly, your blood sugar levels will spike for a long time after eating, and you likely will develop type 2 diabetes and diabetic damage throughout your body because of the resulting high blood sugar levels** – even if, fortuitously, you happen *not* to develop full-blown type 2 diabetes!

**Diabetics have heightened risks for developing cancer, dementia, Alzheimer's Disease, certain kinds of arthritis, and many other conditions.**

Furthermore, <u>excess fat</u> in your body produces extra <u>estrogens</u> that <u>**promote and *encourage* the formation of cancers**</u>! Remember that all of us have cancer in our bodies, as well as opportunistic cancer-causing viruses and other cancer-causing micro-organisms; and **all of these infectious organisms are waiting for a chance to** *start multiplying when your immune system is down* **because of insufficient amounts of exercise, deprivation of deep sleep, imperfect nutrition, too much stress, etc.**

**Note 9:** What is **your <u>ideal body weight</u>?** It is based on **two criteria:** the "pinch" test, and the "beer belly" test when you gently pinch the fat on the front of your abdomen near your belly button while standing erect, and gently pinch all the way down to your abdominal muscles.

Your ideal body weight is

1. the weight at which you realize not more than **about <u>two to two and a half inches</u> of distance between your thumb and your index finger.**

2. Likewise, when you view your stomach from a side view in front of a mirror, **you should *not* have a *beer belly*.** (This is an important criterion because some people have beer bellies, and have less than an inch of fat pinch because all of the *external* belly fat is stretched out!)

If you <u>fail either test individually</u>, you are overweight and very unhealthy – even if you do not feel abnormal.

Thus, losing excess weight is **absolutely critical** to your cancer prevention and cancer reversal program! This and previous chapters amply supply you with all the technical information that you need to succeed! **So, do yourself a favor and fully commit to doing what you need to do!**

Doing a combination exercise program that includes <u>both</u> Interval Training and strength-building exercises will optimize your after-burn calories and BMR, and, hence, your weight loss, once you reach a good level of conditioning. **Your BMR needs to be revved up to optimally burn excess body fat!**

<u>Note 10</u>: <u>Women and Exercise</u>: I have known many dozens of women who, at the beginning of training, complained bitterly about exercising ("always hated gym class," etc.). However, **the majority of these women ultimately became great lovers of exercise once they got over the initial stages of getting in condition, and then started to see results!** In my opinion, this is both a gratifying and interesting phenomenon!!!

This phenomenon may apply also to men, but to a substantially lesser extent. However, I have to admit that I just do not know with 100% certainty if women generally respond more positively than men to good weight loss programs because, over the years, most of my personal training clients have been women! – It would be a great subject for a master's thesis or a PhD dissertation!

**An added benefit of a regular, sufficiently demanding exercise program is <u>healthier skin</u> – with <u>fewer wrinkles</u> and less-deep wrinkles!**

The eight references listed below support the recommendations of this chapter; and the titles of these references aptly describe the subject matter of the studies.

# References

Blair, S.N., & Brodney, S. (1999). Effects of physical inactivity and obesity on morbidity and mortality: Current evidence and research issues.

*Medicine and Science in Sports and Exercise, 31*(11Suppl), S646-S662.

Katzmarzyk, P.T., et al. (2005). Metabolic syndrome, obesity, and mortality: Impact of cardiorespiratory fitness.

*Diabetes Care, 28*, 391-397.

Lee, I.M., & Skerrett, P.J. (2001). Physical activity and all-cause mortality: What is the dose-response relation?

*Medicine and Science in Sports and Exercise, 33*(6 Suppl), S459-S471.

Myers, J., et al. (2004). Fitness versus physical activity patterns in predicting mortality in men.

*American Journal of Medicine, 117*, 912-918.

Oguma, Y., & Shinoda-Tagawa, T. (2004). Physical activity decreases cardiovascular disease risk in women.

*American Journal of Preventive Medicine, 26*(5), 407-418.

Warburton, D. E., Gledhill, N., & Quinney, A. (2001b).

Musculoskeletal fitness and health.

*Canadian Journal of Applied Physiology, 26,* 217-237.

Warburton, D.E., Gledhill, N., & Quinney, A. (2001a). The effects of changes in musculoskeletal fitness and health.

*Canadian Journal of Applied Physiology, 26,* 161-216.

**War**burton, D.E.R., Nicol, C.W., & Bredin, S.S.D. (2006). Health benefits of physical activity: The evidence.

*Canadian Medical Association Journal, 174*(6), 801-809.

# Chapter Seven

# Strength-Building Exercises

⸻ ★ ⸻

The general idea here is to do at least the **bare minimum** of exercises to hit the large muscle groups. Below, the main muscle groups are listed, along with some relevant exercises, and the number of repetitions ("reps") that you should do to the point of muscle failure; that is, you should select a weight or resistance such that you can only do the indicated number of repetitions – and be struggling on the last one or two repetitions. For your "bare minimum" workout, select just one exercise for each muscle group, and aim for <u>at least two workouts per week</u>, and <u>ideally three workouts per week</u> – with one or two days off between workouts. Doing just one exercise for each of the nine muscle groups should take you no more than a total of 20 minutes – and maybe only 15 minutes – once you are fully acclimated!

One concept that you might want to consider is to change-up the exercise that you do for a given muscle group over the course of a week or a month. For example, for your biceps muscles, you might alternate between Bicep Curls and Chin Ups on subsequent workouts.

<u>Note</u>: In the interest of simplicity in the table below, some of the muscles used in a given exercise have been *represented* by just one muscle. For example, the Shoulder Shrug and Chest Press exercises use more than the stated muscles. If someday you should choose to become more schooled in fitness, anatomy, and exercise physiology, you will learn more of the nitty gritty muscle details then.

| **Muscles** | **Exercises** | **# of Reps to "Muscle Failure"** |
|---|---|---|
| **Biceps** | Bicep Curls<br><br>Chin Ups (including weight-assisted machines) | 6 to 10 |
| **Triceps** | Tricep Extensions<br><br>Dips (including weight- assisted machines)<br><br>Chest Press<br><br>Overhead Press | 6 to 10 |

# CANCER

| | | |
|---|---|---|
| **Pecs (chest)** | Pec Flies<br>Chest Press | 6 to 10 |
| **Deltoids (lateral) (shoulders)** | Lateral Raises | 6 to 10 |
| **Deltoids (posterior)** | Seated Row | 6 to 10 |
| **Trapezius (shoulders)** | Shoulder Shrugs | 6 to 10 |

| | | |
|---|---|---|
| **Abdominals** | Abdominal Crunch Machine | 8 to 15 |
| **Quads (front of thighs)** | Leg Presses<br>Leg Extensions | 12 to 15 |
| **Hamstrings (back of thighs)** | Leg Curl Machine (seated or prone version) | 12 to 15 |

# CANCER

## Optimum Order of Exercises

For efficiency of your schedule, you should **do _both_ your cardio and your strength-building exercises in _the same workout_**. Follow the order listed here to maximize your workout results, and *to reduce your risk for injury.*

**First,** do your **upper body strength-building exercises** – that is, for the muscles of your arms, shoulders, chest, and upper back.

**Second,** do your **Interval Training** (cardio) workout.

**Third,** do your **strength-building exercises for the muscles of your core [that is, your lower back, abdomen, and side muscles ("obliques")] and the muscle of your legs.** You can do your core and leg exercises in any order that you like.

# Chapter Eight

# Deep Sleep and the Role of Sunshine

---✦★✦---

Sleep is critical to every facet of your health – even including losing excess weight. It is important is to get a healthy amount of **<u>deep sleep</u> virtually every night**. The amount of sleep that your body needs depends on your genetics – and can vary from one or two sleep cycles (a sleep cycle is about 1.5 hours), to about seven or eight sleep cycles. However, most people will need around 7 to 8 hours of sleep each night. Sleep is a time when your body potentially relaxes in a major way.

In addition, sleep allows

- your body to rejuvenate itself – including "cleaning" your brain of debris
- your immune system to rejuvenate itself
- your brain to solve and/or resolve conflicts and other

problems

- your body to more efficiently lose excess weight
- your brain to plan for the future
- your brain to create new concepts – for such areas as art, marketing, writing, etc.
- your body to release pent-up stress
- your skeletal muscles to recover from your heavy-duty exercise program

Ideally, you should have **no television or computers in your bedroom. In addition, it is wise to allow no land-line phones and no cell phones to be on during sleeping hours, and, preferably, not in the bedroom at all!**

Ideally, you should also have **dark curtains** to keep your bedroom as dark as possible during sleeping hours. You can use one or two (or more) **fans** to provide background noise so that you are less likely to be awakened at night by extraneous, low volume noises. Finally, the **temperature** of your bedroom should be as cool as you like it, or, if your partner likes it cooler, you should go along with their preference and use covers to compensate for the coolness.

Many believe that they can **make up for sleep lost** during the work week by "sleeping in" on the weekend. However, this is a dangerous and major fallacy! **When you habitually skimp on sleep during the work week, your brain is not working optimally.**

Among other things, not only is your brain not sharp, but also you run the risk of <u>falling asleep</u> while driving or at a staff meeting at your job! (That would be embarrassing, wouldn't it? Furthermore, you might be fired if it happened often!) So, use your brain wisely and make the safe, logical lifestyle choice for yourself and your family and friends!

As is implied in one of the studies (Beccuti & Pannain, 2011**), among the many benefits of getting plenty of sleep virtually each night is that you will more easily maintain your ideal body weight!**

In addition, **getting enough deep sleep virtually every night will greatly help <u>reduce your risk of many cancers, type 2 diabetes, heart attacks, and strokes,</u>** as is clear from the titles of many of the references. Of course, getting plenty of exercise and practicing great nutrition will further reduce your risks for these diseases!

Also, check the references in <u>Chapter 23</u> for more on sleep.

## The Role of Sunshine

Many people have a love-hate relationship with sunlight! They love the warmth and cheeriness of it, but hate the effects that it can have on their bodies: increased risk for skin cancers, and premature aging (including wrinkles) of their skin. The following provides a relatively new, positive perspective on sunlight!

**People who get a lot of sunlight (for example, in the summer) have a lower incidence of tuberculosis infection than those who do not get a lot of sunlight – for example, in the winter** (Koh, et al.,

2013). Furthermore, **it is well known that infections in a person's body cause inflammation, which is the starting point for cancers and other pathological conditions to begin to develop.**

**The exact mechanism for this relationship between sunlight and tuberculosis is not yet understood. However, it also is known that exposure to sunlight results in the skin producing nitric oxide (NO)** (Geldenhuys, et al., 2014), which helps to relax arteries, and thus decrease high blood pressure.

Yet another study concludes that **women who get a lot of sunlight have a 30% lower incidence of type 2 diabetes than women who do not get a lot of sunlight exposure** (Lindqvist, et al., 2010). **This is relevant because diabetics have a higher incidence of cancers than non-diabetics, which is due, at least in part, because diabetics have a greater degree of inflammation in their bodies than non-diabetics.**

In addition, **cancer survival rates are better when sunlight exposure is increased** (Lim, et al., 2006).

Thus, ultraviolet radiation from the sun does not fully deserve the criticism that it has received over the years! However, that does NOT mean that you should not work hard to reduce sunlight exposure to your skin – especially areas that tend to get a high exposure, such as your head, neck, and ears; instead, cover these areas as well as you can, and get just a few minutes each sunny day to other areas, for example, your legs. In addition, **some clothes are available that will greatly reduce the amount of UV rays that reach your skin, which is important because ultraviolet rays can penetrate through many clothing materials.**

# References

Ball, L.J., et al. (2016). The pathophysiologic role of disrupted circadian and neuroendocrine rhythms in breast carcinogenesis.

*Endocrine Reviews, 37*(5), 450-466.

Beccuti, G., & Pannain, S. (2011). Sleep and obesity.

*Current Opinion in Clinical Nutrition and Metabolic Care, 14*(4), 402412.

Cho, Y., et al. (2015). Effects of artificial light at night on human health: A literature review of observational and experimental studies applied to exposure assessment.

*Chronobiology International, 32*(9), 1294-1310.

Geldenhuys, S., et al. (2014). Ultraviolet radiation suppresses obesity and symptoms of metabolic syndrome independent of vitamin D in mice fed a high-fat diet.

*Diabetes 63*(11): 3759-3769.

Koh, G.C., et al. (2013). Tuberculosis incidence correlates with sunshine: An ecological 28-year time series study.

*PLoS One 8*(3): e57752 and following.

Lim, H.S., et al. (2006). Cancer survival is dependent on season of diagnosis and sunlight exposure.

*International Journal of Cancer 119*(7): 1530-1536.

Lindqvist, P.G., et al. (2010). Are active sun exposure habits related to lowering risk of type 2 diabetes mellitus in women, a prospective cohort study?

*Diabetes Research and Clinical Practice 90*(1): 109-114.

Mirick, D.K., et al. (2013). Night shift work and levels of 6sulfatoxymelatonin and cortisol in men.

*Cancer Epidemiology, Biomarkers & Prevention, 22*(6), 1079-1087.

Tähkämö, L., et al. (2018). Systematic review of light exposure impact on human circadian rhythm.

*Chronobiology International, 36*(2), 151-170.

# Chapter Nine

# Stress Reduction and Unexpected Sources of Stress to Your Body

------- ★ ★ ★ -------

Unexpected and generally **unrecognized sources of stress** (possibly unrecognized even by many health professionals) are numerous and include the following sources. This list is not exhaustive, but most likely it will open your eyes to sources previously unknown to you.

- *imperfect* **nutrition,** including consuming too much sugar and sugar equivalents
- **a non-optimal or nonexistent cardio exercise program**
- **a non-optimal or nonexistent strength-building exercise program**
- **an imperfect sleep regimen:** that is,
    1. an insufficient amount of *deep* sleep virtually every night,

# CANCER

and/or

2. having to sleep during the day due to a second or third shift job, or lack of self-discipline, and/or lack of a rigid, regular time to go to sleep each night or day

- **holding grudges**

- often **being angry** (particularly in situations in which being more laid back and forgiving would be more appropriate)

- **lack of humility**

- **lack of spirituality** (i.e., not being respectful of your body, your mind, and the minds and bodies of other human beings; and not respecting the environment)

- having **too much stress of any type**

## A Few Tips

1. When stressed out by a large or difficult task or job, one way to decrease your stress is to **break the job down into a series of smaller, more manageable tasks,** and then to determine the optimum or most efficient order in which to do them.

2. <u>Meditation</u> can also greatly help reduce stress. For example, throughout each day, allow yourself to **take** *<u>momentary mental health breaks</u>* (from about 30 seconds to about three minutes) to dream about your favorite vacation spot or some other favorite activity or location. You might also benefit from

decorating the walls of your office and/or home with photographs of special places and people, as well as works of art in general.

3. **Psychotherapy** can also be a beneficial tool to decrease excess stress that you may have in your life. A good psychotherapist will assist you in setting priorities, in seeing aspects of your life in a better perspective, and in how to maneuver and/or change aspects that are not emotionally and therapeutically productive.

4. Another great promoter of stress reduction is **sex. As a result of a sexual climax, the anti-stress (and feel-good) hormone oxytocin is released.** (Oxytocin has other functions in the body – especially in a woman during delivery of a baby.)

5. Another stress reduction technique is to take mental account of tension in your muscles, and *mentally will* **your tense muscles to relax**! With practice, you will find that **you can do your whole body in less than a minute – even in five seconds or less**! This technique may also reduce your blood pressure! (I always do it several seconds before I have my blood pressure taken! For the record, my last blood pressure measurement was 102/58! Not bad for a 75-year-old dude!)

6. If you have been the victim of violent acts (verbal abuse and other emotional abuse, sexual abuse, etc.), you might respond with **unhealthy lifestyle choices,** such as doing drugs and alcohol, gaining excess weight, etc. However, what is key here is to realize that, **if you are reactively abusing yourself,** *you*

are _allowing your abuser to win_!!!

So, think it through, and choose the healthiest life possible so that *YOU are the winner!*

**Important Notes:** When a person is under a high level of stress (especially when the stress is constant or nearly constant!), two things will happen, among many other things!

<u>First,</u> that person **will have a hard time (nearly impossible, sometimes)** <u>learning new subject matter.</u>

<u>Second,</u> that person often will suffer a <u>**drop in the ability to think clearly**</u>. In retrospect regarding a very stressful period in life, you probably will be able to relate to these two major effects of stress as they played out in your life!

These effects of stress are due primarily to **high levels of the stress hormones <u>adrenaline</u> (also known as epinephrine) and <u>cortisol</u>.**

To put this into a practical perspective, **think of what happens to a child who is expected to do well in school when their parents are <u>constantly at war</u>!** Their stress hormones are likely to be so high that they cannot retain material, and they fail to thrive at the very thing that they are working hardest to achieve! So, learning at school decreases, and grades plummet!

# References

———— ★ ★ ★ ————

Aune, D., et al. (2016). Whole grain consumption and risk of cardiovascular disease, cancer, and all cause and cause specific mortality: Systematic review and dose-response meta-analysis of prospective studies.

*British Medical Journal, 353,* i2716 and following.

Beccuti, G., & Pannain, S. (2011). Sleep and obesity.

*Current Opinion in Clinical Nutrition and Metabolic Care, 14*(4), 402412.

Bressan, P., & Kramer, P. (2016). Bread and other edible agents of mental disease.

*Frontiers in Human Neuroscience, 10,* 130 and following.

Emaus, M.J., et al. (2016). Vegetable and fruit consumption and the risk of hormone receptor-defined breast cancer and the EPIC cohort.

*American Journal of Clinical Nutrition, 103*(1), 168-177.

Lauby-Secretan, B., et al. (2016). Body fatness and cancer -- Viewpoint of the IARC Working Group.

*The New England Journal of Medicine, 375*(8), 794-798.

Mirick, D.K., et al. (2013). Night shift work and levels of 6-sulfatoxymelatonin and cortisol in men.

*Cancer Epidemiology, Biomarkers & Prevention, 22*(6), 1079-1087.

Petimar, L., et al. (2019). Dietary index scores and invasive breast cancer risk among women with a family history of breast cancer.

*American Journal of Clinical Nutrition, 109*(5), 1393-1401.

Salo, P., et al. (2014). Work time control and sleep disturbances: Prospective cohort study of Finnish public sector employees.

*Sleep, 37*(7), 1217-1225.

Sternberg, D.A., et al. (2013). The largest human cognitive performance dataset reveals insights into the effects of lifestyle factors and aging. *Frontiers in Human Neuroscience, 7,* 292 and following.

Studte, S., et al. (April 2015). Nap sleep preserves associative but not item memory performance,

*Neurobiology of Learning and Memory, 120,* 84-93.

# Chapter Ten

# Your Mindset

---  ★ ★ ★  ---

Mindset (or attitude) is so important to your overall health, but it alone cannot overcome the absence of knowledgeable, intelligent action on your part. I recommend that you **write down your starting game plan** (**for your desires and goals**) **in a spiral notebook** – including at least **tentative dates** for instituting each of the many phases that you will be experiencing. As you complete each phase, and, if applicable, each sub-phase, check it off your list. (Important Note: **If you do not set dates, you likely are** *just dreaming* **and** *wasting your time!*)

Also, be certain to avoid being totally rigid in your plans so that you have the on-going option to reconsider and reconfigure your plans to optimize your results as you learn more about your body, and about your physical, mental, and spiritual capabilities and desired directions!

# CANCER

Remember:

<u>*With the best mindset, you can do virtually anything*</u>!

One of the best examples (Rosenthal & Jacobsen, 1992) I have ever seen about the power of attitude was carried out by a school district in a very clever, two-part experiment. For the first part, the school system told a group of teachers (who had the worst teaching records in the district) that it had been discovered that "they were the very best teachers in the district." For the second part, the school system told that group of teachers that they would be teaching "the best and the brightest students" (who actually were the worst students) in the district. **The results were amazing: The "worst students" performed well above average, compared to the other supposedly "better" students in the district!**

Think about those results! *The worst* **teachers, teaching** *the worst* **students, but** *yielding the best results!!!* These results speak directly to <u>*the astounding power of mindset*</u>*!!!*

A second example relates to an encounter between a grizzly bear and a grandmother who had a grandchild to protect. The grizzly was clearly intent on feasting on the child, but the grandmother, wielding nothing but a broom, would have nothing of that! With only sheer determination, immense anger, and a fierce <u>*attitude* that she **would prevail**</u>**,** she showed no fear and warded off the grizzly! You might wonder if the grizzly admitted its wimpiness to other grizzlies in the area! How could the grizzly not have realized that it had the strength to wipe out the grandmother with only a gentle swipe with one of its humongous paws?

# Reference

Rosenthal, R. & Jacobson, L. (1992). *Pygmalion in the classroom: teacher expectation and pupils' intellectual development* (Newly expanded Edition). Bancyfelin,

Carmarthen, Wales: Crown House Pub. ISBN 9781904424062

# Chapter Eleven

# Avoid Drugs, Smoke, Smoking, and Alcohol!

———————— ★ ★ ★ ————————

There is no need to beat around the bush and use a lot of words.

Simply: **<u>Do not smoke anything</u> (no cigarettes, e-cigarettes, cigars, marijuana, or any other inhalable carcinogenic substances).** And try to **avoid being in confined quarters** (house, car, office, restaurant, bar, etc.) **where you would be subjected to second-hand smoke.** Also, do your best to **avoid** *third-hand smoke,* **which means avoiding areas in which smokers have smoked and left residue from smoke;** such situations have been shown to increase cancer and asthma risks for other residents of the house. Such third hand smoke deposits cancer-causing residues on furniture, on clothes, on rugs, etc. Thus, smokers who try to *"do good"* by only smoking outdoors **still cause <u>more than 4,000 toxins and heavy metals</u> (including lead, arsenic, cadmium, etc.) in tobacco smoke to be spread throughout the living quarters, and increase the risks for cancers, asthma, and cardiovascular and other diseases for those living there.

If you smoke long enough, and live long enough, you will likely die after a prolonged, agonizing death from <u>COPD</u> (Chronic Obstructive Pulmonary Disease), in which you will drown from fluid in your lungs. Furthermore, no amount of narcotics will be capable of easing your extreme pain brought on by COPD – 24/7/365! **The time over which such *slow death* will occur can vary <u>from many months to many years</u>!**

Finally, **it is unfortunate that so many smokers are heavily addicted – especially in view of the fact that <u>hypnosis</u> and <u>acupuncture</u> are quite effective in reversing such addictions** (Chen. P., et al., 2018; Lynn, S.J., et al., 2010; Motlagh, S.L., et al., 2016; Munson, S.O., et al., 2018; Shin, N.Y., et al., 2017; Wu, S.L., et al., 2016).

## The Extra Danger for the Diabetic Who Smokes

As noted above, the 4,000-plus poisons in cigarettes increase the risk for cancer in people who smoke. What is not as widely known is that **<u>diabetic smokers have an even greater risk of contracting cancer</u> than those who are not diabetic.** However, this should not be a surprise because **a diabetic is not healthy, which means that their immune system is not fully functional to fight the million-plus viruses, etc., that, every day, are trying to establish footholds from which cancers will develop!**

The references cited below support the above conclusions.

Furthermore, <u>*ALL smoke is damaging to your lungs*</u> – be it smoke from a campfire, from a fireplace, or from a forest fire! So, for example, if you are around a campfire, position yourself up-wind from the fire.

**Drugs are <u>SO scary</u> and <u>SO dangerous!</u> Do not use illegal drugs or misuse legal drugs.** On any given day, you do not know how your body will respond to a particular drug. For example, **you could suffer a fatal heart attack on your first use of cocaine, or on the thousandth use;** and no one can tell you when such an unfortunate event might befall you! Also, **the use of drugs will <u>greatly decrease the level of function of your immune system</u>, which means that your body will be <u>much more susceptible to developing many of the common cancers</u>,** as well as some of the not-so-common cancers! Furthermore, <u>**your actual brain size will decrease, as well as your IQ**</u>! Use your God-given brain, and **do <u>not</u> give in to the temptation to** *"be cool"* with your *so-called friends!*

## Alcohol

You should consider alcoholic drinks to be drugs, too. **When alcohol that you have consumed reaches your liver, it is converted immediately to acetaldehyde, which is a potent carcinogen.** State-of-the-art research concludes that <u>**no amount of alcohol consumption is "safe."**</u>

Finally, you probably have seen ads on TV for prescription drugs that can have side effects such as "infections" and/or "cancers." Realize **that <u>all</u> drugs with these possible side effects are**

**diminishing the functioning of the patient's immune system.** If your physician prescribes one of these drugs to you, you should ask her/him if the drug is absolutely necessary, or if there is a less immune damaging drug available!

# References

Bagnardi, V., et al. (2013). Light alcohol drinking and cancer: A meta-analysis.

*Annals of Oncology, 24*(2), 301-308.

Bonelli, L., et al. (2003). Exocrine pancreatic cancer, cigarette smoking, and diabetes mellitus: a case-control study in northern Italy.

*Pancreas, 27*(2), 143-149.

Burton, R. & Sheron, N. (2018). No level of alcohol consumption improves health.

*The Lancet, 392*(10152), 987-988.

Cao, Y., et al. (2015). Light to moderate intake of alcohol, drinking patterns, and risk of cancer: Results from two prospective US cohort studies.

*British Medical Journal, 351*, h4238 and following.

Chen, P., et al. (2018). Acupuncture for alcohol use disorder.

*International Journal of Physiology, Pathophysiology and Pharmacology, 10*(1), 60-69.

Connor, J., et al. (2017). Alcohol-attributable cancer deaths under 80 years of age in New Zealand.

*Drug and Alcohol Review, 36*(3), 415-423.

Giovannucci, E., et al. (2010). Diabetes and cancer: A consensus report.

*CA: A Cancer Journal for Clinicians, 60*(4), 207-221.

Huxley, R., et al. (2005). Type-II diabetes and pancreatic cancer:

A meta-analysis of 36 studies.

*British Journal of Cancer, 92,* 2076-2083.

Kadlecová, P., et al. (2015). Alcohol consumption at midlife and risk of stroke during 43 years of follow-up: Cohort and twin analyses. *Stroke, 46*(3), 627-623.

Klein, W.P., et al. (2020). Alcohol and cancer risk. Clinical and research implications.

*Journal of the American Medical Association, 323*(1), 23-24.

Knott, C.S., et al. (2015). All-cause mortality and the case for age specific alcohol consumption guidelines: Pooled analyses of up to 10 population-based cohorts.

*British Medical Journal, 350,* h 384 and following.

Larsson, S.C., et al. (2005). Overall obesity, abdominal obesity, diabetes and cigarette smoking in relation to the risk of pancreatic cancer in two Swedish population-based cohorts.

*British Journal of Cancer, 93*, 1310-1315.

Leibson, C.L., et al. (2005). Probability of pancreatic cancer following diabetes: A population-based study.

*Gastroenterology, 129*(2), 504-511.

Le Marchand, L., et al. (1997). Associations of sedentary lifestyle, obesity, smoking, alcohol use, and diabetes with the risk of colorectal cancer.

*Cancer Research, 57*(21), 4787-4794.

Lindemann, K., et al. (2008). Body mass, diabetes and smoking, and endometrial cancer risk: A follow-up study.

*British Journal of Cancer, 98*, 1582-1585.

Linhart, K., Bartsch, H., & Seitz, H.K. (2014). The role of reactive oxygen species (ROS) and cytochrome P-450 2E1 in the generation of carcinogenic etheno-DNA adducts.

*Redox Biology, 3*, 56-62.

Lowenfels, A.B., & Maisonneuve, P. (2006). Epidemiology and risk factors for pancreatic cancer.

*Best Practice & Research Clinical Gastroenterology, 20*(2), 197-209.

Luo, J., et al. (2007). Body mass index, physical activity and the risk of pancreatic cancer in relation to smoking status and history of diabetes: A large-scale population-based cohort study in Japan – The LPHC study.

*Cancer Causes & Control, 18*(6), 603-612.

Lynn, S.J., et al. (2010). Hypnosis and smoking cessation: The state of the science.

*American Journal of Clinical Hypnosis, 52*(3), 177-181.

Millonig, G., et al. (2011). Ethanol-mediated carcinogenesis in the human esophagus implicates CYP2E1 induction and the generation of carcinogenic DNA-lesions.

*International Journal of Cancer, 128*(3), 533-540.

Motlagh, F.E., et al. (2016). Acupuncture therapy for drug addiction.

*Chinese Medicine, 11,* 16 and following.

Munson, S.O., et al. (2018). Ability of hypnosis to facilitate movement through stages of change for smoking cessation.

*International Journal of Clinical and Experimental Hypnosis, 66*(1), 58-62.

Pandeya, N., et al. (2015). Cancers in Australia attributable to the consumption of alcohol.

*Australian and New Zealand Journal of Public Health, 39*(5), 408-413.

Passarelli, M.N., et al. (2016). Cigarette smoking before and after breast cancer diagnosis: Mortality from breast cancer and smoking-related diseases.

*Journal of Clinical Oncology, 34*(12), 1315-1322.

Petticrew, M., et al. (2018). How alcohol industry organisations mislead the public about alcohol and cancer.

*Drug and Alcohol Review, 37*(3), 293-303.

Rimm, E.B., et al. (1995). Prospective study of cigarette smoking, alcohol use, and the risk of diabetes in men.

*British Medical Journal, 310,* 555 and following.

Scheideler, J.K. & Klein, W.M.P. (2018). Awareness of the link between alcohol consumption and cancer across the world.

*Cancer Epidemiology, Biomarkers & Prevention, 27*(4), 429-437.

Shin, N.Y., et al. (2017). Acupuncture for alcohol abuse disorder: A meta-analysis.

*Evidence-Based Complementary and Alternative Medicine, 2017,* 7823278 and following.

Suzuki, R., et al. (2005). Alcohol and postmenopausal breast cancer risk defined by estrogen and progesterone receptor status: A prospective cohort study.

*Journal of the National Cancer Institute, 97*(21): 1601-1608.

Wood, A.M., et al. (2018). Risk thresholds for alcohol consumption: Combined analysis of individual-participant data for 599,912 current drinkers in 83 prospective studies.

*The Lancet, 391*(10129), 1513-1523.

Wu, S.L., et al. (2016). Acupuncture for detoxification in

treatment of opioid addiction.

*East Asian Archives of Psychiatry, 26*(2), 70-76.   **[A review.]**

# Chapter Twelve

# Type 2 Diabetes and the Increased Risk for Cancers in General

★ ★ ★

Type 2 diabetics have long been known to be at an increased risk for cancers (de Beer & Liebenberg, 2014, Fernandez, et al., 2001; Rabøl, et al., 2009a; Aroor, et al., 2012; Rabøl, et al., 2009b; Huang, 2009; Zeigler-Johnson, et al., 2013; Huang, et al., 2014; Rhee, et al., 2019). What is so unfortunate about this correlation is that type 2 diabetes is preventable more than 90% of the time, and also reversible over 90% of the time. [Actually, type 2 diabetes is preventable and reversible probably around 95% of the time!] Thus, both the diabetes and the cancer are highly preventable, or at least have highly limited odds of development when well-researched principles are practiced. Data on the effects of high blood sugar levels on the risk of type 2 diabetes have been known for years. (Fernandez, et al.,2001; Rabøl, et al., 2009a; Aroor, et al., 2012; Rabøl, et al., 2009b; Huang, 2009; Zeigler-Johnson, et al., 2013; Huang, et al., 2014; Rhee, et al., 2019). Furthermore, **Zeigler-Johnson, et al., 2013** addresses baldness, which is caused by high blood sugar levels, and which correlates with an increased risk for contracting cancer!

In a nutshell, you will find that **the combination of *Interval Training* for the exercise portion of your reversal protocol, plus excellent nutrition, is highly effective in achieving this objective. Also, you will greatly improve your odds of success by incorporating** *strength-building exercise* **into the mix and getting a sufficient amount of deep sleep virtually every night.**

On the nutrition front, you should **eat lots of fruits, vegetables, nuts and seeds, and** *totally* **eliminate mammalian meat, processed meats, deep fried foods, and food loaded with sugar and/or** *sugar equivalents,* such as **food made of flour of any kind** (for example, all pastas, breads, crackers, pretzels, cakes, pie crusts, pastries, and other similar foods), as well as the inner pulp of potatoes (the skin is where almost all of the healthy nutrients reside).

Furthermore, as a diabetic, <u>when you eat fruits (fresh or frozen), be sure to eat them as part of an all-around healthy meal</u> in order to limit the size of the rise in your blood glucose level that follows naturally after eating – whether or not you are diabetic!

Another nutrition tip is to **eat two or three servings of nuts before eating your breakfast, your lunch, and your dinner.** One serving of nuts is one ounce, which is equivalent to 18 to 20 pistachio nut kernels without their shells. **When you regularly follow this protocol, you will experience smaller rises in your blood glucose levels – compared to the rise you would have had without the nuts.** (Moreira Alves, et al., 2014; Del Gabb, et al., 2015; Yu, et al., 2016;

Weng, et al., 2016; Luu, et al., 2015).

Finally, **increase the quality of your nutrition by** *adding variety* **in** *all* **of the food groups: fruits, vegetables (ideally including beans, lentils, greens, etc.), nuts, and seeds.** You should also greatly limit your intake of fats and oils, which are large sources of excess calories; there are exceptions, such as foods like **avocados and olives,** which **are loaded with very healthy fats.**

**Yet another reason to cure your type 2 diabetes is that your chances of getting dementia, including Alzheimer's disease, are greatly increased if you do not** (Moreira, 2013; Biesels, et al., 2005; Watson & Craft, 2003; Swaminathan & Jicha, 2014). Remember that

**Curing your type 2 diabetes only requires you to adopt a healthy <u>lifestyle</u> with respect to nutrition, exercise, stress, and sleep!**

# References

---- ★ ★ ★ ----

Aroor, A., et al. (2012). Mitochondria and oxidative stress in the cardiorenal metabolic syndrome.

*Cardiorenal Medicine, 2*(2), 87- 198.

Biesels, G.J., et al. (2005). Increased risk of Alzheimer's disease in Type II diabetes: Insulin resistance of the brain or insulin-induced amyloid pathology?

*Biochemical Society Transactions, 33*(Pt 5),1041-1044.

de Beer, J.C., & Liebenberg, L. (2014). Does cancer risk increase with HbA1c, independent of diabetes?

*British Journal of Cancer, 110*(9), 2361-2368.

Del Gabb, L.C., et al. (2015). Effect of tree nuts on blood lipids, apolipoproteins, and blood pressure: Systematic review, meta-analysis, and dose-response of 61 controlled intervention studies.

*American Journal of Clinical Nutrition, 102*(6): 1347-1356.

Fernandez-Real, J.M., et al. (2001). Circulating interleukin 6 levels, blood pressure, and insulin insensitivity in apparently healthy men and women.

# CANCER

*The Journal of Clinical Endocrinology & Metabolism, 86*(3), 11541159.

Huang, P.L. (2009). A comprehensive definition for metabolic syndrome.

*Disease Models & Mechanisms, 2*(5-6), 231-237.

Huang, Y., et al. (2014). Prediabetes and the risk of cancer: A meta-analysis.

*Diabetologia, 57*(11), 2261-2269.

Luu, H.N., et al. (2015). Prospective evaluation of nut/peanut consumption with total and cause-specific mortality.

*JAMA Internal Medicine, 175*(5), 86-96.

Moreira Alves, R.D., et al. (2014). High-oleic peanuts: New perspective to attenuate glucose homeostasis disruption and inflammation related to obesity.

*Obesity (Silver Spring, MD),22*(9),1981-1988.

Moreira, P.I. (2013). High-sugar diets, type 2 diabetes and Alzheimer's disease.

*Current Opinion in Clinical Nutrition and Metabolic Care, 16*(4), 440445.

Rabøl, R. et al. (2009a). Effect of hyper glycemia on mitochondrial respiration in type 2 diabetes.

*The Journal of Clinical Endocrinology & Metabolism, 94*(4), 1372-1378.

Rabøl, R., et al. (2009b). Improved glycemic control decreases inner mitochondrial membrane leak in type 2 diabetes.

*Diabetes, Obesity and Metabolism, 11*(4), 355-360.

Rhee, H., et al. (2019). Metabolic syndrome and prostate cancer: A review of complex interplay amongst various endocrine factors in the pathophysiology and progression of prostate cancer.

*Hormones & Cancer, 7*(2), 75-83

Sun, M.K., & Alkon, D.L. (2006). Links between Alzheimer's disease and diabetes.

*Drugs of Today (Barcelona, Spain), 42*(7), 481-489.

Swaminathan, A., & Jicha, G.A. (2014). Nutrition and prevention of Alzheimer's dementia.

*Frontiers in Aging Neuroscience, 6*, 282 and following.

Tsilidis, K.K., et al. (2015). Type 2 diabetes and cancer umbrella review of meta-analyses of observational studies.

*British Medical Journal, 350*, g7607 and following.

Watson, G.S., & Craft, S. (2003). The role of insulin resistance in the pathogenesis of Alzheimer's disease: Implications for treatment.

*CNS Drugs, 17*(1), 27-45.

Weng, Y.Q., et al. (2016). Association between nut consumption and coronary heart disease.

*Coronary Artery Disease, 27*(3), 227-232.

# CANCER

Yu, Z., et al. (2016), Association between nut consumption and inflammatory biomarkers.

*American Journal of Clinical Nutrition, 104(3), 722-728.*

Zeigler-Johnson, C., et al. (2013). Relationship of early-onset baldness to prostate cancer in African American men.

*Cancer Epidemiology, Biomarkers & Prevention, 22(4), 589-596.*

# Chapter Thirteen

# Avoiding Noxious Fumes (Gasoline, Vehicle Emissions, Formaldehyde), Asbestos, and Other Environmental Hazards

★ ★ ★

You might feel that you bear the brunt of numerous unhealthy chemicals as you go about your daily life – and to the detriment of your health. Unfortunately, you are probably right! This chapter will provide you with some food for thought for your fears. Hopefully, this chapter will alert you to a few sources that you might not have considered. We would be happy to write more on this subject here, but it would take many encyclopedias-worth of material to cover the millions of dangerous chemicals that potentially could harm your health – from chemicals in foods and plants, to chemicals in the environment (defined to include sources outside, as well as inside homes and buildings, and even in cosmetics), etc.!

# CANCER

Try to **avoid *all* fumes from gasoline. For example, put yourself *upwind* when filling your vehicle's gas tank;** and, if you regularly engage in walking or running on a sidewalk or on the side of a road, try to avoid doing so during rush hours, and also see if there are any available routes with less traffic.

<u>Gasoline</u> **contains *benzene* to boost its octane rating. Benzene is a well-known, very potent carcinogen. It is just *one of the many dangerous components of gasoline* and of vehicle exhaust** (a product of gasoline combustion to drive pistons and wheels)! You should also do your best to avoid or minimize breathing diesel exhaust.

Another source of noxious fumes is the smell that you experience when you breathe the air near a photocopy machine. Additionally, you should avoid exposure to <u>*formaldehyde*</u> (for example, from illegal flooring from China), and vapors from many glues and from some paints. Formaldehyde also gives new cars part of their *new car smell!* Therefore, **when you purchase a new car, drive with the windows down until the smell disappears.** In addition, the odor of some laundry detergents can smell noxious. Generally, **if an odor *smells* <u>toxic</u>, be safe and take the conservative approach of doing your utmost to avoid, or greatly lessen, your exposure to that odor.**

<u>Nail polish</u> and nail polish remover typically contain acetone – another known carcinogen; so, use them only in a very well-ventilated area!

In 2018, Monsanto was ordered by the judge in the trial to pay over $289 million dollars to a groundskeeper who developed non-Hodgkin's lymphoma as a result of using Monsanto's weed killer

**in his job over a period of two and a half years.** In the trial, secret internal documents of Monsanto showed that Monsanto had known for decades about the dangers of its product **Roundup™,** and knowingly used dishonest, illegal tactics to conceal those dangers. Therefore, this is another product that you should avoid at all costs!

Another mega-corporation, Johnson & Johnson, recently recalled 33,000 bottles of baby powder due to the possibility of asbestos contamination (Hsu & Rabin, 2019). Unfortunately, talcum often occurs in nature with asbestos!

Yet another study, based in Taiwan, recently reported an association between the use of hair dyes and prostate cancer (Tai, et al., 2016).

Also, **there is a risk of contracting cancer from using your cell phone – particularly if you use it "glued to your ear" for large amounts of time each day** (Benson, V.S., et al. 2013; Hardell, L., et al. 2007; Kesari, S., et al. 2013; Myung, S-K., et al. 2009; Repacholi, M.H., et al. 2012; Teo, C., et al. 2009)!

In addition, have you ever thought about the health consequences of breathing air that has "rubber dust" from vehicle tires as their treads wear down?

Finally, as noted herein in Chapter One, you probably have seen prescription drug ads on TV, the Internet, etc., in which warnings are posted that taking the given drug carries a risk of infections and/or cancers! If your doctor prescribes one of these drugs, be sure to ask her/him if there is a less dangerous option!

# CANCER

There are other sources of carcinogens that many are not aware of, including many in the health professions – namely, cancer-causing agents in some topical creams, ointments, and underarm deodorants.

For other sources of environmental pollution, see the References below.

# References

Andersen, A., et al. (1999). Work-related cancer in Nordic countries.

*Scandinavian Journal of Work, Environment & Health, 25* Suppl 2, 1-116.

Aragonés, N., et al. (2002). Stomach cancer and occupation in Sweden: 1971-89.

*Occupational & Environmental Medicine, 59*(5), 329-337.

Benson, V.S., et al. (2013). Mobile phone use and risk of brain neoplasms and other cancers: Prospective study.

*International Journal of Epidemiology, 42*(3), 792-802.

Bourdrel, T., et al. (2017). Cardiovascular effects of air pollution.

*Archives of Cardiovascular Diseases, 110*(11), 634-642.

Brannick. K,E., et al. (2012). Prenatal exposure to low doses of bisphenol A increases pituitary proliferation and gonadotroph number in female mice offspring at birth.

*Biology of Reproduction, 87*(4), 82 and following.

Brunekreef, B., et al. (2009). Effects of long-term exposure to traffic-related air pollution on respiratory and cardiovascular mortality in the Netherlands: The NLCS-AIR study.

*Research Report (Health Effect Institute), 139,* 5-71.

Callahan, C.L., et al. (2018). Lifetime exposure to air pollution and methylation of tumor suppressor genes in breast tumors.

*Environmental Research, 161,* 418-424.

Caprino, L., & Togna, G.I. (1998). Potential health effects of gasoline and its constituents: A review of current literature (1990-1997) on toxicological data.

*Environmental Health Perspectives, 106*(3),115 - 125.

Chen, W., et al. (2019). Disparities by province, age, and sex in site-specific cancer burden attributable to 23 potentially modifiable risk factors in China: A comparative risk assessment.

*Lancet Global Health, 7*(2), e257-e269.

Eckstrum, K.S., et al. (2018). Effects of exposure to the endocrine disrupting chemical bisphenol A during critical windows of murine pituitary development.

*Endocrinology, 159*(1), 119-131.

Egeghy, P.P., et al. (2000). Environmental and biological monitoring of benzene during self-service automobile refueling.

*Environmental Health Perspectives, 108*(12), 1195-1202.

Gaudet, M.M., et al. (2019). Blood levels of cadmium and lead in relation to breast cancer risk in three prospective cohorts.

*International Journal of Cancer, 143*(10), 2380-2389.

Gawda, A., et al. (2017). Air pollution, oxidative stress, and exacerbation of autoimmune diseases.

*Central European Journal of Immunology, 42*(3), 305-312.

Grohs, M.N., et al. (2019). Prenatal maternal and childhood bisphenol A exposure and brain structure and behavior of young children.

*Environmental Health, 18*(1), 85 and following.

Hardell, L., et al. (2007). Long-term use of cellular phones and brain tumours: Increased risk associated with use for ≥ 10 years.

*Occupational & Environmental Medicine, 64*(9), 626-632.

Hsu, T., & Rabin, C. (October 18, 2019). Johnson & Johnson recalls baby powder over asbestos worry.

*The New York Times.*

Huebner, W.W., et al. (2000). Incidence of lymphohematopoietic malignancies in a petrochemical industry cohort: 1983-94 follow up.

*Occupational & Environmental Medicine, 57*(9), 605-614.

Joshi, A.D., et al. (2012). Fish intake, cooking practices, and risk of prostate cancer: Results from a multi-ethnic case-control study.

*Cancer Causes & Control, 23*(3), 405-420.

Joshi, A.D., et al. (2012). Red meat and poultry, cooking practices, genetic susceptibility and risk of prostate cancer: Results from a multiethnic case-control study.

*Carcinogenesis, 33*(11), 2108-2118.

Joshi, A.D., et al. (2015). Meat intake, cooking methods, dietary carcinogens, and colorectal cancer risk: Findings from the Colorectal Cancer Family Registry.

*Cancer Medicine, 4*(6), 936-952.

Kesari, S., et al. (2013). Swedish review strengthens grounds for concluding that radiation from cellular and cordless phones is a probable human carcinogen.

*Pathophysiology, 20*(2), 123-129.

Kjaerheim, K. (1999). Occupational cancer research in the Nordic countries.

*Environmental Health Perspectives, 107* (Suppl 2), 233-238.

Kiriluk, K.J., et al. (2012). Bladder cancer risk from occupational and environmental exposures.

*Urologic Oncology: Seminars and Original Investigations, 30*, 199-211.

Lee, D-H. (2018). Evidence of the possible harm of endocrine-disrupting chemicals in humans: Ongoing debates and key issues.

*Endocrinology and Metabolism (Seoul), 33*(1), 44-52.

Lehmler, H.-J., et al. (2018). Exposure to bisphenol A, bisphenol F, and Bisphenol S in U.S. adults and children: The National Health and Nutrition Examination Survey 2013-2014.

*ACS Omega, 3*(6), 6523-6532.

Lin, P.H., et al. (2015). Nutrition, dietary interventions and prostate cancer: The latest evidence.

*BMC Medicine, 13*, 3 and following.

Lipworth, L., et al. (2009). Epidemiologic characteristics and risk factors for renal cell cancer.

*Clinical Epidemiology, 1*, 33-43.

Liu, J., et al. (2018). Exposure and dietary sources of bisphenol A (BPA) and BPA-alternatives among mothers in the APrON cohort study.

*Environment International, 119*, 319-326.

Lynge, E., et al. (1997). Risk of cancer and exposure to gasoline vapors.

*American Journal of Epidemiology, 145*(5), 449-458.

Matuszczak, E., et al. (April 10, 2019). The impact of bisphenol A on fertility, reproductive system, and development: A review of the literature.

*International Journal of Endocrinology, 2019*, 4068717 and following.

McNabola, A., et al. (2007). Optimal cycling and walking speed for minimum absorption of traffic emissions in the lungs.

*Journal of Environmental Science and Health Part A, Toxic/Hazardous Substances & Environmental Engineering, 42*(13), 1999-2007.

Meeker, J.D. (2012). Exposure to environmental endocrine disruptors and child development.

*Archives of Pediatrics & Adolescent Medicine, 166*(6), E1-E7.

Morgan, M., et al. (2017). Environmental estrogen-like endocrine disrupting chemicals and breast cancer.

*Molecular and Cellular Endocrinology, 457,* 89-102.

Myung, S-K., et al. (2009). Mobile phone use and risk of tumors: A meta-analysis.

*Journal of Clinical Oncology, 27*(33), 5565-5572.

Nie, J., et al. (2007). Exposure to traffic emissions throughout life and risk of breast cancer: The Western New York Exposure and Breast Cancer (WEB) study.

*Cancer Causes & Control, 18*(9), 947-955.

Piazza, M.J., & Urbanetz, A.A. (2019). Environmental toxins and the impact of other endocrine disrupting chemicals in women's reproductive health.

*JBRA Assisted Reproduction, 23*(2), 154-164.

Powell, J.B., & Ghotbaddini, M. (2014). Cancer-promoting and inhibiting effects of dietary compounds: Role of the aryl hydrocarbon receptor (AhR).

*Biochemical Pharmacology, 3*(1), 10.4172/2167.

Preciados, M., et al, (2016). Estrogenic endocrine disrupting chemicals influencing NRF1 regulated gene networks in the development of complex human brain diseases.

*International Journal of Molecular Sciences, 17*(12), pii: E2086 and following.

Raaschou-Nielsen, O., et al. (2011). Air pollution and cancer incidence: A Danish cohort study.

*Environmental Health: A Global Access Science Source, 10,* 67 and following.

Rahbar, M.H., et al. (2017). Environmental exposure to dioxins, dibenzofurans, bisphenol A, and phthalates in children with and without autism spectrum disorder living near the Gulf of Mexico.

*International Journal of Environmental Research and Public Health, 14*(11), 1425 and following.

Ramadan, N., et al. (2018). Disruption of neonatal cardiomyocyte physiology following exposure to bisphenol-A.

*Scientific Reports, 8*(1), 7356 and following.

Repacholi, M.H., et al. (2012). Systematic review of wireless phone use and brain cancer and other head tumors.

*Bio Electro Magnetics, 33*(3), 187-206.

# CANCER

Rivollier, F, et al (2019). Perinatal exposure to environmental endocrine disruptors in the emergence of neurodevelopmental psychiatric diseases: A systematic review.

*International Journal of Environmental Research and Public Health, 16*(8), 1318 and following.

Rochester, J. (2013). Bisphenol A and human health: A review of the literature.

*Reproductive Toxicology, 42,* 132-155.

Rodgers, K.M., et al. (2018). Environmental chemicals and breast cancer: an updated review of epidemiological literature informed by biological mechanisms.

*Environmental Research, 160,* 152-182.

# Chapter Fourteen

# Late Evening Eating Restrictions Eliminate and Reduce Cancer Risks

⸻ ★ ★ ★ ⸻

A 2016 study showed that "prolonged nightly fasting" reduced the risk of breast cancer recurrence in women. The authors suggested that their conclusion might be the result of improved blood glucose regulation and improved sleep (Marinac, et al., 2016).

The scientists studied 2,413 women aged 27 to 70 years (average age 52.4 years) at the time of their breast cancer diagnosis. They found that women who had a 12.5-hour or more break between dinner and breakfast had a lower risk of breast cancer recurrence than those who had less than a 12.5-hour break. Also, those with a longer break had lower values for hemoglobin A1c, which reflects the "average" blood glucose level for the previous two months. In other words, **taking longer breaks between one's dinner and breakfast the following morning (specifically, longer than 12.5 hours) produces lower spikes in blood sugar and/or shorter**

# CANCER

durations for the after-eating blood sugar levels; thus, although blood sugar rises normally after eating, one's blood sugar level rises to a healthier level when this regimen is followed.

A similar study in mice produced essentially the same results. (Chung, et al., 2016).

# References

Bandin, C., et al. (2015). Meal timing affects glucose tolerance, substrate oxidation and circadian-related variables: A randomized, crossover trial.

*International Journal of Obesity (London), 39(5), 828-833.*

Chung, H., et al. (2016). Time-restricted feeding improves insulin resistance and hepatic steatosis in a mouse model of postmenopausal obesity.

*Metabolism, 65(12), 1743-1754.*

Del Gabbo, L.C., et al. (2015). Effect of tree nuts on blood lipids, apolipoproteins, and blood pressure: Systematic review, meta-analysis, and dose-response of 61 controlled intervention studies.

*American Journal of Clinical Nutrition, 102(6): 1347-1356.*

Kogevinas, M., et al. (2018). Effect of mistimed eating patterns on breast and prostate cancer risk (MCC-Spain Study).

*International Journal of Cancer, 143(10), 2380-2389.*

Luu, H.N., et al. (2015). Prospective evaluation of the association of nut/peanut consumption with total and cause-specific mortality.

*JAMA Internal Medicine, 175*(5), 755-766.

Marinac C.R.., et al. (2016). Prolonged nightly fasting and breast cancer prognosis.

*JAMA Oncology, 2*(8), 1049-1055.

Moreira Alves, R.D., et al. (2014). High-oleic peanuts: New perspective to attenuate glucose homeostasis disruption and inflammation related to obesity.

*Obesity (Silver Spring, Md), 22*(9), 1981-1988.

Weng, Y.Q., et al. (2016). Association between nut consumption and coronary heart disease: A meta-analysis.

*Coronary Artery Disease, 27*(3), 227-232.

Yu, Z., et al. (2016). Association between nut consumption and inflammatory biomarkers. *American Journal of Clinical Nutrition, 104*(3), 722-728.

# Chapter Fifteen

# Support Groups Online

In this, the Digital Age, it is not surprising that online support groups have sprung up on the Internet. The first such large scale entity in this domain is www.colontown.org, which was cofounded on Facebook in 2016 by Erika Hanson Brown; it has over 40 *secret* groups on Facebook.

At age 58, Brown was diagnosed with advanced colorectal cancer. She was cured and has remained disease free for over 16 years. She cofounded Colontown to fill a variety of needs:

- in general, to provide support groups for cancer patients
- to provide a website (in addition to the websites of NIH and the National Cancer Institute) where cancer patients can learn about ongoing clinical trials, many of which still have open slots for cancer patients who want to be research subjects
- to provide a platform on which cancer patients can communicate with other cancer patients – often forming deep,

# CANCER

lasting relationships

- to provide a platform on which patients with other disease states can benefit in the same way as patients in the above three bullet points

A relatively simple enrollment form is available, as is a phone helpline: **877-422-2030.**

Colontown has stimulated a few other sites with similar features and capabilities, and many more are likely to spring up in the coming months and years. Just checkout related hits when you do a Google search.

# Chapter Sixteen

# The Weakest Link Concept

---  ★ ★ ★  ---

The Weakest Link Concept is perhaps the simplest concept herein. This is true because, when it comes to your health, you truly are no better than your weakest area.

For example, **if you are a smoker, there is no way that you can have a fully healthy body – even if it is just one cigarette a day!** Of course, the amount of damage to your body will be dose-dependent; thus, on a more-or-less sliding scale, the amount of damage will depend on how many cigarettes you smoke in a day.

Similarly, **nutrition deficits and the lack of a sufficient quantity of appropriately demanding exercise every week will produce real, negative, and obvious repercussions;** just consult the previous chapters for specifics on research publications!

One of the unfortunate truths is that all the areas covered so far in this book are <u>silent killers</u> – meaning that **there may be ZERO palpable effects from <u>not</u> practicing great health!** A similar effect has been noted for decades by the medical profession relative to high blood pressure; **a person can have an elevated blood pressure and never have any overt, recognizable symptom!** That is why high blood pressure is known as **"the silent killer,"** and why you should have your blood pressure checked every month or so! Consider using the blood pressure measuring machines that are in many grocery stores.

In the weakest link concept, a relevant conclusion is that **those who refuse to exercise the health practices outlined in this book are not acting in their fullest spiritual manner; that is, <u>they cannot honestly assert that they are acting as highly spiritual beings with respect to their own bodies</u>!**

# Chapter Seventeen

# Fitness and Longevity: What Does it REALLY Mean for You?

★ ★ ★

IN 1999, the first large scale study was published that showed that the more fit a person is, the more likely they are to live longer than the unfit person. (Wei, M., et al. 1999). This large study was necessary so that – at least from a statistical aspect – the data would be irrefutable. Since then, many other studies have further solidified this conclusion. However, the important point is: **What do these data really show?** In other words, **to what critical conclusions do these data speak that are very relevant to, and beneficial for, YOUR overall health?**

If you have read every word in this book up to this point, then the answer to this question will come as no surprise:

- **Your odds of having stellar health and living a long, fulfilling life are great!**
- **Your odds of being or becoming a type 2 diabetic are close**

to nil.

- Your odds of having or developing any of the various cardiovascular diseases is very low [that is, risks for heart attacks, strokes, peripheral artery disease, metabolic syndrome (also known as Syndrome X), etc.]
- Your odds of having significant mental health issues (that is, deep depression, feelings of low self-worth, and an array of other mental disorders and/or illnesses) is small.
- Your odds of having or developing many of the common cancers is greatly reduced.
- Your odds of suffering from osteoporosis are reduced, as are your odds of breaking bones.
- Your odds of experiencing osteoarthritis (and some other kinds of arthritis) are reduced.
- Your odds of experiencing renal (kidney) failure are lessened, as are your odds of needing hemodialysis or a renal transplant.
- Your odds of being immobile (for example, largely confined to a bed or wheelchair) are reduced.

This list could go on and on . . . However, in short, YOUR **OVERALL HEALTH** is what is at stake!

If your current level of health is not at its peak, do not despair. The odds are that <u>you can improve your health at any age</u>! – It REALLY is that simple!!!

Just use this book as your roadmap!

# References

Aune, D., et al. (2015). Body mass index, abdominal fatness and the risk of gallbladder disease.

*European Journal of Epidemiology, 30*(9), 1009-1019.

Aune, D., et al. (2016). BMI and all-cause mortality: Systematic review and non-linear dose-response meta-analysis of 230 cohort studies with 3.74 million deaths among 30.3 million participants.

*British Medical Journal, 353,* i2156 and following.

Bhaskaran, K., et al. (2014). Body mass index and risk of 22 specific cancers: A population-based cohort study of 5.24 million UK adults. *Lancet, 384*(9945), 755-765.

Bodai, B.I., et al. (2018). Lifestyle medicine: A brief review of its dramatic impact on health.

*The Permanente Journal, 22,* 17-25.

Friedenreich, C.M., et al. (2016). Physical activity and survival after prostate cancer.

*European Urology, 15,* 1241-1245.

Gerritsen, J., et al. (2016). Exercise improves quality of life in patients with cancer: A systematic review and meta-analysis of randomized controlled trials.

*British Journal of Sports Medicine, 50,* 796-803

Kabat, G.C., et al. (2015). Risk of breast, endometrial, colorectal, and renal cancers in postmenopausal women in association with a body shape index and other anthropometric measures.

*Cancer Causes and Control, 26(2),* 219-229.

Keimling, M., et al. (2014). The association between physical activity and bladder cancer: A systematic review and meta-analysis.

*British Journal of Cancer, 110,* 1862-1870.

Kenfield, S.A., et al. (2016). Development and application of a lifestyle score for prevention of lethal prostate cancer.

*Journal of the National Cancer Institute, 108(3),* dvj329 and following.

Krautkramer, K.A., et al. (2017). Chemical signaling between gut microbiota and host chromatin.

*Journal of Biological Chemistry, 292(21),* 8582-8593.

Lauby-Secretan, B., et al. (2016). Body fatness and cancer – viewpoint of the IARC Working Group.

*The New England Journal of Medicine, 375,* 794-798.

Moghaddam, A.A., et al. (2007). Obesity and risk of colorectal cancer: A meta-analysis of 31 studies with 70,000 events.

*Cancer Epidemiology, Biomarkers & Prevention, 16*(12), 2533-2547.

Oke, S., & Martin, A. (2017). Insights into the role of the intestinal microbiota in colon cancer.

*Therapeutic Advances in Gastroenterology, 10*(5), 417-428.

Pernar, C.H., et al. (2018). A prospective study of the association between physical activity and the risk of prostate cancer defined by clinical features and TMPRSS2:ERG.

*European Urology, 76*(1), 33- 40.

Thomas, R.J., et al. (2017). Exercise-induced biochemical changes and their influence on cancer: A scientific review.

*British Journal of Sports Medicine, 51*(8), 640-644.

Wei, M., et al. (1999). Relationship between low cardiorespiratory fitness and mortality in normal weight, overweight, and obese men.

*Journal of the American Medical Association, 282*(16), 1547-1553.

# Chapter Eighteen

## Spirituality and Giving Back

---  ★ ★ ★ ---

As mentioned earlier, the foundation for spirituality is respect for all life. Thus, the highly spiritual person makes time to share their talents with people in need. Giving back to people in need might include befriending someone who is being bullied, befriending a lonely senior citizen, and so many more acts of unselfish kindness. Someone who works in the healthcare field, or in the teaching field, is able to "kill two birds with one stone" by earning a salary and also helping others to the best of their abilities.

**A most interesting observation is that a person who helps others in need often receives as much benefit as the receiver of the help – and, many times, even more!**

Getting outside of oneself allows a person to avoid the tendency toward a more-or-less self-centered life, and, thus, ensuring a happier, more fulfilled life! Frequently, another important byproduct of lending a helping hand is <u>**stress reduction**</u>!

<u>The bottom line</u>: **Things will come together and align optimally in your life when you follow the prescriptions laid out in this book!**

# Chapter Ninteen

## Miscellany – A Note on Cleanliness

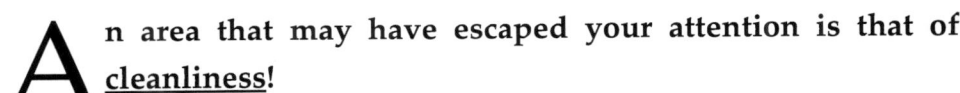

An area that may have escaped your attention is that of <u>cleanliness</u>!

Have you ever been in a house, office, or business in which the floor was full of dust bunnies? Whether there is substantial accumulation of "regular" dust on one surface or another, or large dust bunnies that usually occur only on floors, **the dust likely contains carcinogens!** The only effective tactic to get around this is to <u>clean, clean, clean</u>!

Perhaps you are familiar with the expression

**Cleanliness is Next to Godliness!**

Now you know a major reason why!

# References

Balaram, P., et al. (2002). Oral cancer in southern India: The influence of smoking, drinking, paan-chewing and oral hygiene.

*International Journal of Cancer, 98,* 440-445.

Hamilton, K., et al. (2017). Examining the relationship between park neighborhoods, features, cleanliness, and condition with observed weekday park useage and physical activity: A case study.

*Journal of Environmental and Public Health, 2017,* Article ID 7582402, 11 pages.

Lucak, A., et al. (June, 2018). The prevalence of the most important risk factors associated with cervical cancer.

*Materia Sociomedica,* 30( 2), 131-135.

Nelson, A. (August, 2014). Rules to practice by: Safety first and cleanliness is close to…

*Contraceptive Technology,* August, 2014.

Wakefield-Rann, R., et al. (2018). "It's just a never-ending battle": The role of hygiene ideals and the dynamics of everyday life in constructing indoor ecologies.

*Human Ecology Review, 24(2),* 61-80.

# Chapter Twenty

# The Holy Trinity of Un-Healthy

———————— ★ ★ ★ ————————

Cancer is a terrifying topic to most people; and they often are even more terrified when they learn that cancer and cancer producing viruses (and other carcinogenic micro-organisms, too) have been in their bodies from birth!!!

The implication of this realization: **You need to do everything possible to reduce your risks in the first place! To go one step further, you need to recognize the enormous job that your immune system does every second of every day to protect you from infections and millions of "wanna-be" cancers!**

These concepts remind me of a saying that I have modified slightly:

**Prevention Is Always the Best CURE!**

One of the focuses and objectives of this book is to make you aware that you have many options, and – now that you know and understand those options – that you should institute ALL of them as soon as you possibly can!

Another focus and objective of this book is to make you aware of the new field of **epigenetics,** and how you can use it to **deactivate negative, unhealthy genes in your cells, and activate healthy genes in your cells.** Thus, for example, if you are a female who happens to have both of the breast cancer-promoting genes, BRCA1 and BRCA2, you can greatly decrease your odds of developing breast cancer by following the prescriptions in this book! This concept is fully applicable to other cancers, too!

"The Trinity of Un-Health" refers to **the three main culprits** that **produce the majority of unhealthiness in the world:**

- **Overweightness** and **Inactivity** (or, at least an insufficient level and amount of exercise),
- **Poor nutrition** (or, at least very imperfect nutrition), and
- **An insufficient amount of deep sleep virtually every night,** and/or irregular sleep hours, or working nightshifts and sleeping during the day.

The All-Important Bottom Line:

**YOU, and ONLY YOU, have the immense power to control your destiny!** When you "live right," an amazingly beneficial cascade of events will transpire:

- Your overall somatic (physical) health will be incredibly

better!

- Your **mental health will be much better**, including being happier, feeling more fulfilled, and being much less likely to experience depression and other mental deficiencies!

- **You will be much more energetic**

- **You will have healthier, more positive attitudes**

- You will be **more efficient** and **more directed** in virtually every aspect of your life!

- If you are a student (of any age!), you will find **yourself more easily absorbing new material and concepts** than ever before!

- **You will be much <u>more spiritual</u>, including getting outside of yourself to help others who are in need!**

- You will experience **more friendships, and <u>deeper relationships</u>**!

- Your primary care physician might wonder why you "visit" his/her office less often than you used to, and **how you <u>transformed yourself</u>**!

- You will come to understand, first-hand, that

"Your Health Is Your Wealth!

And that, indeed, you are

QUITE WEALTHY!"

# SECTION II

### The WHY: Why Certain Lifestyle Choices are Healthy or Unhealthy

# Chapter Twenty-One

# Why Being Overweight is ALWAYS Unhealthy

---★ ★ ★---

A slew of studies unequivocally shows that, if you are overweight, you are unhealthy because **your excess fat increases inflammation throughout your body**, and this, in turn, increases your risks for heart attacks, strokes, metabolic syndrome (Syndrome X), Peripheral Artery Disease, Type 2 diabetes, cancer, and dementia, including Alzheimer's! Also, the latest research shows that being **even a small amount overweight is unhealthy** (Okada, et al., 2016) – thus dispelling the earlier belief that being slightly overweight was healthy: the earlier studies had a major flaw in their design. In addition, **beneficial results from cardio exercise can be realized in just six weeks** (Manukka, et al., 2018)! (**Actually, in my practice as a Personal Trainer, I have seen strong cardio results for clients in less than two weeks with interval training!**)

When you are overweight, **your excess fat secretes estrogen,** which <u>promotes the growth of cancers</u> in your body, and also <u>promotes inflammation</u> (the two are interrelated)!

Furthermore, **when you are overweight, other <u>inflammatory markers</u> are circulating throughout your entire body** (a partial list):

- C-reactive protein (CRP)
- High-sensitivity C-reactive protein (hs-CRP)
- interleukin-6 (IL-6)
- tumor necrosis factor receptor 2 (TNFR2)
- insulin
- TNF-alpha (a measure of cell damage in your body)
- insulin-like growth factors
- serum amyloid A (SAA), and many more!

To put all of this into perspective, just remember that **<u>inflammation is the starting point for cancers, arterial plaque (clots), and a host of other ailments</u>**, including some kinds of arthritis! Obviously, you do not want your entire body to be vulnerable to life-threatening diseases and conditions! – And the danger is proportional to how overweight you are!

# References

---- ★★★ ----

Bailargeon, J., & Rose, D.P. (2006). Obesity, adipokines and prostate cancer (Review).

*International Journal of Oncology, 28* (3), 737-745.

Becker, S., Dossus, L., & Kaaks, R. (2009). Obesity related hyperinsulinaemia and hyperglycaemia and cancer development.

*Archives of Physiology and Biochemistry,115*(2), 86-96.

Bhaskaran, K., et al. (2014). Body-mass index and risk of 22 specific cancers: A population-based cohort study of 5.24 million UK adults. *Lancet, 384*(9945), 755-765.

Boeing, H., et al. (2012). Critical review: Vegetables and fruit in the prevention of chronic diseases.

*European Journal of Nutrition, 51*(6), 637-663.

[Note: This excellent review contains 298 references.]

Ellulu, M.S., et al. (2016). Obesity can predict and promote systemic inflammation in healthy adults.

*International Journal of Cardiology, 215,* 318-324.

Fernandez-Real, J.M., et al. (2001). Circulating interleukin 6 levels, blood pressure, and insulin sensitivity in apparently healthy men and women.

*Journal of Clinical Endocrinology & Metabolism, 86*(3), 1154-1159.

Ford, C.T., et al. (2016). Identification of (poly)phenol treatments that modulate the release of pro-inflammatory cytokines by human lymphocytes.

*The British Journal of Nutrition, 115*(10), 1699-1710.

Fridlender, M., et al. (2015). Plant derived substances with anti-cancer activity: From folklore to practice.

*Frontiers in Plant Science, 6,* 799 and following.

Fukumura, D., et al. (2016). Obesity and cancer: An angiogenic and inflammatory link.

*Microcirculation, 23*(3), 191-206.

Gati, A., et al. (2014). Obesity and renal cancer. Role of adipokines in the tumor-immune system conflict.

*Oncoimmunology, 39* (1), e27810 and following.

[NOTE: This article reviews the multitude of factors and concepts that apply to understanding <u>how obesity contributes to cancer in kidneys</u>. The same principles also apply to most – if not all – other tissues in the body.]

Hayes, B.D., et al. (2016). Exercise and prostate cancer: Evidence and proposed mechanisms for disease modification.

# CANCER

*Cancer Epidemiology, Biomarkers and Prevention, 25*(9), 1281-1288.

Huffman, D.M., et al. (2013). Abdominal obesity, independently from caloric intake, accounts for the development of intestinal tumors in Apc1638N/+ female mice.

*Cancer Prevention Research, 6*(3), 177-187.

Incio, J., et al. (2016). Obesity-induced inflammation and desmoplasia promote pancreatic cancer progression and resistance to chemotherapy.

*Cancer Discovery, 6*(8), 852-869.

Jiang, Y., et al. (2016). A sucrose-enriched diet promotes tumorigenesis in mammary gland in part through the 12-lipoxygenase pathway.

*Cancer Research, 76*(1), 24-29.

Johannson, I., et al. (2018). Dairy intake revisited – Associations between dairy intake and lifestyle related cardiometabolic risk factors in a high milk consuming population.

*Nutrition Journal, 17*(1), 110 and following

Kendall, B.J., et al. 2015. Cancers in Australia in 2010 attributable to overweight and obesity.

*Australian and New Zealand Journal of Public Health, 39*(5), 452-457.

Key, T.J. (2011). Fruit and vegetables and cancer risk.

*British Journal of Cancer, 104*(1), 6-11.

Key, T.J., & Spencer, E.A. (2007). Carbohydrates and cancer: An overview of the epidemiological evidence.

*European Journal of Clinical Nutrition, 61* (Suppl 1), S112-S121.

Koeth, R.A., et al. (2013). Intestinal microbiota metabolism of L-carnitine, a nutrient in red meat, promotes atherosclerosis.

*Nature Medicine, 19*(5): 576-585.

Lin, P.H., et al. (2015). Nutrition, dietary interventions and prostate cancer: The latest evidence.

*BMC Medicine 13*: 3 and following.

[This review article summarizes studies that show the effect of nutrition on prostate cancer. From 197 references, these authors concluded that **a healthy dietary pattern** **consists of consuming lots of fruits and vegetables, and consuming very limited quantities of refined carbohydrates, total fat, saturated fats, and cooked red meats** (that is, meat from mammals)].

Lu, W., et al. (2016). Dairy products intake and cancer mortality risk: A meta-analysis of 11 population-based cohort studies.

*Nutrition Journal, 15*(1), 91 and following.

Melkonian, S.C., et al. (2016). Glycemic index, glycemic load, and lung cancer risk in non-Hispanic whites.

*Cancer Epidemiology, Biomarkers & Prevention, 25*(3), 532-539.

Michaëlsson, K., et al. (2017). Milk, fruit and vegetable, and total antioxidants intakes in relation to mortality rates: Cohort studies in women and men.

*American Journal of Epidemiology, 185*(5), 345-361.

Michaëlsson, K., et al. (2014). Milk intake and risk of mortality and fractures in women and men: Cohort studies.

*British Medical Journal, 349,* g6105 and following

Moghaddam, A.A., Woodward, M., & Huxley, R. (2007). Obesity and risk of colorectal cancer: A meta-analysis of 31 studies with 70,000 events.

*Cancer Epidemiology, Biomarkers & Prevention, 16*(12), 2533-2547.

Mourouti, N., et al. (2017). Optimizing diet and nutrition for cancer survivors: A review. *Maturitas, 105,* 33-36.

Munukka, E., et al. (2018). Six-week endurance exercise alters gut metagenome that is not reflected in systemic metabolism in overweight women.

*Frontiers in Microbiology, 9,* 2323 and following.

Nunez, C., et al. (2018). Physical activity, obesity and sedentary behavior and the risks of colon and rectal cancers in the 45 and up study.

*BMC Public Health, 18*(1), 325 and following.

Okada, R., et al. (2016). Upper-normal waist circumference is a risk marker for metabolic syndrome in normal-weight subjects.

*Nutrition, Metabolism & Cardiovascular Diseases, 26*(1), 67-76.

O'Keefe, S.J., et al. (2015). Fat, fiber and cancer risk in African Americans and rural Africans.

*Nature Communications, 6*, 6342 and following.

**[This study shows that switching from pro-inflammatory, unhealthy nutrition to healthy nutrition produces a significant <u>lowering of risk factors for colon cancer in just 2 weeks</u>!]**

Parikesit, D., et al. (2016). The impact of obesity towards prostate diseases.

*Prostate International, 4*(1), 1-6.

Peppa, M., & Raptis, S.A. (2008). Advanced glycation end products and cardiovascular disease.

*Current Diabetes Reviews, 4*(2), 92-100. [Note:

**[This study shows that advanced glycation end products (AGEs) <u>increase inflammation</u>, and thereby increase the risk for cardiovascular diseases. However, it is now also known that <u>inflammation (and AGEs) independently increase the risk for developing cancers in general</u>.]**

Reinisalo, M., et al. (2015). Polyphenol stilbenes: Molecular mechanisms of defense against oxidative stress and aging-related diseases.

*Oxidative Medicine and Cellular Longevity, 2015*, 340520 and following.

Rhee, H., Vela, I., & Chung, E. (2016). Metabolic syndrome and prostate cancer: A review of complex interplay amongst various endocrine factors in the pathophysiology and progression of prostate cancer.

*Hormones & Cancer, 7*(2), 75-83.

Rose, D.P., Gracheck, P.J., & Vona-Davis, L. (2015). The interactions of obesity, inflammation and insulin resistance in breast cancer.

*Cancers (Basel), 7*(4), 2147-2168.

Rundle, A., et al. (2013). Obesity and future prostate cancer risk among men after an initial benign biopsy of the prostate.

*Cancer Epidemiology, Biomarkers & Prevention, 22*(5), 898-904.

Shah, R.V., et al. (2016). Abdominal fat radiodensity, quantity and cardiometabolic risk: *The Multi-Ethnic Study of Atherosclerosis.*

*Nutrition, Metabolism & Cardiovascular Diseases, 26*(2), 114-122.

Shah, S.C., et al. (2018). Microbial-host interactions in inflammatory bowel disease, obesity and obesity-related metabolic disease.

*Gastroenterology, 155*(5), 1283-1286.

Short, K.R., et al. (2009). Vascular health in children and adolescents: Effects of obesity and diabetes.

*Vascular Health and Risk Management, 5,* 973-990.

Silva, S.A., et al. (2015). Prostate hyperplasia caused by long-term obesity is characterized by high deposition of extracellular matrix and increased content of MMP-9 and VEGF.

*International Journal of Experimental Pathology, 96(1), 21-30.*

Sinha, R., et al. (2009). Meat intake and mortality: A prospective study of over half a million people.

*Archives of Internal Medicine, 169(6), 562-571.*

**[<u>Note</u>: This study shows that consuming <u>red meat</u> (which may be taken to mean mammalian meat) and processed meat increases the risks for cancer, cardiovascular diseases, and <u>early death</u>.]**

Sluijs, I., et al. (2010). Dietary intake of total, animal, and vegetable protein and risk of type 2 diabetes in the European Prospective Investigation into Cancer and Nutrition (EPIC)-NL Study. *Diabetes Care, 33(1), 43-48.*

Solfrizzi, V., et al. (2011). Diet and Alzheimer's disease risk factors or prevention: The current evidence.

*Expert Review of Neurotherapeutics, 11(5), 677-708.*

Thomson, C.A., et al. (2014). Nutrition and physical activity cancer prevention guidelines, cancer risk, and mortality in the women's health initiative.

*Cancer Prevention and Research (Philadelphia), 7(1), 42-53.*

Uribarri, J., et al. (2010). Advanced glycation end products in foods, and a practical guide to their reduction in the diet.

*Journal of the American Dietetic Association, 110(6), 911-916.*

Vivante, A., et al. (2012). Body mass index in 1.2 million adolescents and risk for end-stage renal disease.

*Archives of Internal Medicine, 172*(21), 1644-1670.

**[Note: This study shows that overweight adolescents are at an increased risk for both diabetic and non-diabetic end-stage renal disease; thus, they are at an increased risk of requiring hemodialysis for the rest of their lives or needing kidney transplants. However, if they have kidney transplants, but do not make the needed lifestyle changes, they are highly likely to experience end-stage renal disease again.]**

Wagner, M., Steinskog, E.S.S., & Wiig, H. (2015). Adipose tissue macrophages: The inflammatory link between obesity and cancer?

*Expert Opinions on Therapeutic Targets, 19*(4), 527-538.

Weigl, J., Hauner, H., & Hauner, D. (2018). Can nutrition lower the risk of recurrence in breast cancer?

*Breast Cancer (Basel), 13*(2), 86-91.

Yu, E., et al. (2017). Weight history and all-cause and cause-specific mortality in three prospective cohort studies.

*Annals of Internal Medicine, 166*(9), 613-620.

Zheng, H., et al. (2015). Metabolomics investigation to shed light on cheese as a possible piece in the French paradox puzzle.

*Journal of Agricultural and Food Chemistry, 63*(10), 2830-2839.

Zuchetto, A., et al. (2016). Dietary inflammatory index and

prostate cancer survival.

*International Journal of Cancer, 139*(11), 2398-2404.

# Chapter Twenty-Two

# Why Being Sedentary is Always Unhealthy

---★---

If you lack a healthy amount of exercise, you will have unhealthy inflammation with respect to the same factors, and the same effects, as mentioned above in Chapter 21.

In addition, with a sedentary lifestyle, your body will experience (though you will not feel it) **a shortening of telomeres.**

**Telomeres are strands of DNA that protect your chromatin from unraveling. The function of telomeres can be likened to the plastic mini tubes (caps) that encircle the ends of shoelaces.**

They are on the ends of the chromatin (on your DNA – deoxyribonucleic acid) that is in your cells. A related increase in the activity of the enzyme telomerase increases the length of the chromatin end caps when you practice a regular exercise program that is sufficiently demanding, have great nutrition, and get a sufficient amount of deep sleep virtually every night.

The reason you might want to be concerned about telomere end caps is that **lengthy telomeres and increased telomerase activity predict how long you are likely to live,** and may also contribute to your quality of life in ways not yet understood.

A recent study stresses the importance of exercise for your best health (Lee, et al., 2019). Another study shows the beneficial effect of cardio exercise on gut microbiota (Munukka, et al., 2018). (See also Pernar, et al., 2018). Likewise, the other references address the importance of being physically fit to increase the odds of preventing various cancers.

# References

Abbott, S.E., et al. (2016). Recreational physical activity and ovarian cancer risk in African American women.

*Cancer & Medicine, 5*(6), 1319-1327.

Behrens, G., et al. (2014). The association between physical activity and gastroesophageal cancer: systematic review and meta-analysis.

*European Journal of Epidemiology, 29*(3), 151-170.

Cannioto, R., et al. (2016). Chronic recreational inactivity and epithelial ovarian cancer risk: Evidence from the Ovarian Cancer Association Consortium.

*Cancer Epidemiology, Biomarkers & Prevention, 25*(7), 1114-1124.

Cannioto, R.A., & Moysich, K.B. (2015). Epithelial ovarian cancer and recreational physical activity: A review of the epidemiological literature and implications for exercise.

*Gynecological Oncology, 137*(3), 559-573.

Chih, H., et al. (2013). Sitting time, physical activity and cervical intraepithelial neoplasia in Australian women: A preliminary investigation.

*Health Promotion Journal of Australia, 24*(3), 219-223.

Devin, J.L., et al. (2015). The influence of high-intensity compared with moderate-intensity exercise training on cardiorespiratory fitness and body composition in colorectal cancer survivors: A randomised controlled trial.

*Journal of Cancer Survivorship: Research and Practice, 10*(3), 467-479.

Friberg, E., Mantzoros, C.S., & Wolk, A. (2006). Physical activity and risk of endometrial cancer: A population-based prospective cohort study.

*Cancer Epidemiology, Biomarkers & Prevention, 15*(11), 2136-2140.

Friedenreich, C.M., & Cust, A.E. (2008). Physical activity and breast cancer risk: impact of timing, type and dose of activity and population subgroup effects.

*British Journal of Sports Medicine, 42*(8), 636-647.

Friedenreich, C.M., & Orenstein, M.R. (2002). Physical activity and cancer prevention: Etiologic evidence and biological mechanisms.

*Journal of Nutrition, 132*(11 Suppl), 3456S-3464S.

Giovannucci, E.L., et al. (2005). A prospective study of physical activity and incident and fatal prostate cancer.

*Archives of Internal Medicine, 165*(9), 1005-1010.

Hamer, J., & Warner, E. (2017). Lifestyle modifications for patients with breast cancer to improve prognosis and optimize overall health.

*Canadian Medical Association Journal, 189*(7), E268-E274.

Hashemi, S.H.B., et al. (2014). Lifestyle changes for prevention of breast cancer.

*Electronic Physician, 6*(3), 894-905.

Haydon, A.M., et al. (2006). Effect of physical activity and body size on survival after diagnosis with colorectal cancer.

*Gut, 55*(1), 62-67.

Hibler, E. (2015). Epigenetics and colorectal neoplasia: The evidence for physical activity and sedentary behavior.

*Current Colorectal Cancer Reports, 11*(6), 388-396.

Kim, G.H., et al. (2016). Higher physical activity is associated with increased attentional network connectivity in the healthy elderly.

*Frontiers in Aging Neuroscience, 8*, 198 and following.

Lahart, I.M., et al. (2015). Physical activity, risk of death and recurrence in breast cancer survivors: A systematic review and meta-analysis of epidemiological studies.

*Acta Oncologica (Stockholm, Sweden), 54*(5), 635-654.

Lahmann, P.H., et al. (2007). Physical activity and breast cancer:

The European prospective investigation into cancer and nutrition.

*Cancer Epidemiology, Biomarkers & Prevention, 16(1),36-42.*

Lee, D.H., et al. (2019). Association of type and intensity of physical activity with plasma biomarkers of inflammation and insulin response.

*International Journal of Cancer, 145(2), 360-369.*

Lee, J.K., et al. (2013). Mild obesity, physical activity, calorie intake, and the risks of cervical intraepithelial neoplasia and cervical cancer.

*PLoS One, 8(6), e66555 and following.*

Lynch, B.M., et al. (2011). Associations of objectively assessed physical activity and sedentary time with biomarkers of breast cancer risk in postmenopausal women: Findings from NHANES (2003-2006).

*Breast Cancer Research and Treatment, 130(1), 183-194.*

McClellen, J.L., et al. (2014). Exercise effects on polyp burden and immune markers in the ApcMin+ mouse model of intestinal tumorigenesis.

*International Journal of Oncology, 45(2), 861-868.*

Meyerhardt, J.A., et al. (2006). Physical activity and survival after colorectal cancer diagnosis.

*Journal of Clinical Oncology, 24(22), 3527-3534.*

Munukka, E., et al. (2018). Six-week endurance exercise alters gut metagenome that is not reflected in systemic metabolism in overweight women.

*Frontiers in Microbiology, 9,* 2323 and following.

Murphy, E.A., et al. (2011). Benefits of exercise training on breast cancer progression and inflammation in C3(1)SV40Tag mice.

*Cytokine, 55*(2), 274-279.

Murphy, E.A., Enos, R.T., & Velázquez, K.T. (2015). Influence of exercise on inflammation in cancer: Direct effect or innocent bystander?

*Exercise and Sport Sciences Reviews, 43*(3), 134-142.

Olsen, C.M., et al. (2015). Cancers in Australia in 2010 attributable to insufficient physical activity.

*Australian and New Zealand Journal of Public Health, 39*(5), 458-463.

Olsen, C.M., Bain, C.J., Jordan, S.J., Nagle, C.M., Green, A.C., Whiteman, D.C., Webb, P.M., & Australian Cancer Study Group. (2007). Recreational physical activity and epithelial ovarian cancer:

A case-control study, systematic review, and meta-analysis.

*Cancer Epidemiology, Biomarkers & Prevention, 16*(11), 2321-2330.

Pernar, C.H., et al. (2018). A prospective study of the association between physical activity and risk of prostate cancer defined by clinical features and TMPRSS2:ERG.

*European Urology, 76*(1), 33- 40.

Sanchez, N.F., et al. (2012). Physical activity reduces risk for colon polyps in a multiethnic colorectal cancer screening population.

*BMC Research Notes, 5,* 312 and following.

Shah, R.V., Murthy, V.L., & Lima, J.A. (2016). Fitness and coronary artery calcification – reply.

*JAMA Internal Medicine, 176*(5), 716- 717.

Singh, S., et al. (2014). Physical activity is associated with reduced risk of gastric cancer: A systematic review and meta-analysis.

*Cancer Prevention Research (Philadelphia, PA), 7*(1), 12-22.

Singh, S., et al. (2014). Physical activity is associated with reduced risk of esophageal cancer, particularly esophageal adenocarcinoma: A systematic review and meta-analysis.

*BMC Gastroenterology, 14,* 101 and following.

Slattery, M.L. (2004). Physical activity and colorectal cancer.

*Sports Medicine (Aukland, New Zealand), 34*(4), 239-252.

Szender, J.B., et al. (2016). Impact of physical inactivity on risk of developing cancer of the uterine cervix: A case-control study.

*Journal of Lower Genital Tract Disease, 20*(3), 230-233.

Tardon, A., et al. (2005). Leisure-time physical activity and lung cancer: A meta-analysis.

# CANCER

*Cancer Causes & Control, 16*(4), 389-397.

Tehard, B., et al. (2006). Effect of physical activity on women at increased risk of breast cancer: Results from the E3N cohort study.

*Cancer Epidemiology, Biomarkers & Prevention, 15*(1), 57-64.

Thune, I., & Furberg, A.S. (2001). Physical activity and cancer risk: Dose-response and cancer, all sites and site-specific.

*Medicine and Science in Sports and Exercise 33*(6 Suppl): S530-S550.

Voskuil, D.W., Monninkhof, E.M., Elias, S.G., Vlems, F.A., van Leeuwen,F.E., & Task Force Physical Activity. (2007). Physical activity and endometrial cancer risk, a systematic review of current evidence.

*Cancer Epidemiology, Biomarkers & Prevention, 16*(4), 639-648.

Wallace, L., et al. (2018). Relationship between frailty and Alzheimer's disease biomarkers: A scoping review.

*Alzheimer's and Dementia (Amsterdam), 10,* 394-401.

Wei, M., et al. (1999). Relationship between low cardiorespiratory fitness and mortality in normal-weight, overweight, and obese men.

*Journal of the American Medical Association, 282*(16), 1547-1553.

Willis, B.L., et al. (2012). Midlife fitness and the development of chronic conditions in later life.

*Archives of Internal Medicine, 172*(17), 1333-1340.

Zhu, Z., et al. (2012). Effects of energy restriction and wheel running on mammary carcinogenesis and host systemic factors in a rat model.

*Cancer Prevention Research (Philadelphia, PA), 5(3), 414-422.*

# Chapter Twenty-Three

## Why Not Getting Enough Deep Sleep Virtually Every Night is Always Unhealthy

---------- ★ ★ ★ ----------

Many believe that they can make up for sleep lost during the work week by "sleeping in" on the weekend. However, this is a dangerous and major fallacy! When you habitually skimp on sleep during the work week, your brain is not working optimally. Among other things, not only is your brain not sharp, but also you run the risk of falling asleep while driving or at a staff meeting at your job! (That would be embarrassing, wouldn't it? Furthermore, you might be fired if it happened often!) So, use your brain wisely and make the safe, logical lifestyle choice for yourself and your family and friends!

As is implied in one of the studies (Beccuti & Pannain, 2011), among the many benefits of getting plenty of sleep virtually each night is that you will more easily maintain your <u>ideal body weight</u>!

In addition, **getting enough deep sleep virtually every night will greatly help <u>reduce your risk of many cancers, type 2 diabetes, heart attacks, and strokes</u>,** as is clear from the titles of many of the references. Of course, getting plenty of exercise and practicing great nutrition will further reduce your risks for these diseases!

# References

Ayas, N.T., et al. (2003). A prospective study of self-reported sleep duration and incident diabetes in women.

*Diabetes Care, 26(2), 389- 384.*

Ball, L.J., et al. (2016). The pathologic role of disrupted circadian and neuroendocrine rhythms in breast carcinogenesis.

*Endocrine Reviews, 37(5), 450-466.*

Blask, D.E., et al. (2002). Melatonin as a chronobiotic/anticancer agent: Cellular, biochemical, and molecular mechanisms of action and their implications for circadian-based cancer therapy.

*Current Topics in Medicinal Chemistry, 2(2), 113-132.*

Brandin, C., et al. (2015). Meal timing affects glucose tolerance, substrate oxidation and circadian-related variables: A randomized, crossover trial.

*International Journal of Obesity (London), 39(5), 828-833.*

Costas, L., et al. (2016). Night shift work and chronic lymphocytic leukemia in the MCC-Spain case-control study.

*International Journal of Cancer, 139(9), 1994-2000.*

Davis S., & Mirick, D.K. (2006). Circadian disruption, shiftwork and the risk of cancer: A summary of the evidence and studies in Seattle.

*Cancer Causes & Control, 17*(4), 539-545.

Kakizaki, M., et al. (2008). Sleep duration and the risk of breast cancer: The Ohsaki Cohort Study.

*British Journal of Cancer, 99*(9), 1502-1505.

Kim, T.W., et al. (2015). The impact of sleep and circadian disturbances on hormones and metabolism.

*International Journal of Endocrinology, 2015,* 591729 and following.

Kubo, T., et al. (2006). Prospective cohort study of the risk of prostate cancer among rotating-shift workers: Findings from the Japan collaborative cohort study.

*American Journal of Epidemiology, 164*(6), 649-655.

Lamia, K.A. (2017). Ticking time bombs: Connections between circadian clocks and cancer.

*F 1000Research, 6,* 1910 and following.

Lawson, K.A., et al. (2007). Multivitamin use and risk of prostate cancer in the National Institutes of Health-AARP Diet and Health Study.

*Journal of the National Cancer Institute, 99*(10), 754-764.

Mah, C.D., et al. (2011). The effects of sleep extension on the athletic performance of collegiate basketball players.

*Sleep, 34*(7), 943-950.

Minett, G.M., & R Duffield, R. (2014). Is recovery driven by central or peripheral factors? A role for the brain in recovering following intermittent-sprint exercise.

*Frontiers in Physiology, 5,* 24 and following.

Morris, C.J., et al. (2015). Endogenous circadian system and circadian misalignment impact glucose tolerance via separate mechanisms in humans.

*Proceedings of the National Academy of Sciences, 112*(17),

E2225-E2234.

Padmanabhan, K., & Billaud, M. (2017). Desynchronization of circadian clocks in cancer: A metabolic and epigenetic connection.

*Frontiers in Endocrinology, 8,* 136 and following.

Papantoniou, K., et al. (2015). Night shift work, chronotype and prostate cancer risk in the MCC-Spain case control study.

*International Journal of Cancer, 137*(5), 1147-1157.

Passos, G.S., et al. (2011). Effects of moderate aerobic exercise training on chronic primary insomnia.

*Sleep Medicine, 12*(10), 1018- 1027.

Pinheiro, S.P., et al. (2006). A prospective study on habitual duration of sleep and incidence of breast cancer in a large cohort of women.

*Cancer Research, 66*(10), 5521-5525.

Qian, J., & Scheer, F.A. (2016). Circadian system and glucose metabolism: Implications for physiology and disease.

*Trends in Endocrinology and Metabolism, 27*(5), 282-293.

Reid, K.J., et al. (2010). Aerobic exercise improves self-reported sleep and quality of life in older adults with insomnia.

*Sleep Medicine, 11*(9), 934-940.

Reszka, E., et al. (2017). Circadian gene variants and breast cancer.

*Cancer Letters, 390,* 137-145.

Reszka, E., et al. (2018). Circadian gene methylation in rotating-shift nurses: A cross-sectional study.

*Chronobiology International, 35*(1), 111-121.

Salo, P., et al. (2014). Work time control and sleep disturbances: Prospective cohort study of Finnish public sector employees.

*Sleep, 37*(7), 1217-1225.

Schernhammer, E.S., et al. (2003). Night-shift work and risk of colorectal cancer in the nurses' health study.

*Journal of the National Cancer Institute, 95*(11), 825-828.

Schernhammer, E.S., et al. (2001). Rotating nightshifts and risk of breast cancer in women participating in the nurses' health study.

*Journal of the National Cancer Institute, 93*(20), 1563-1568.

Shilts, J., et al. (2018). Evidence for widespread dysregulation of circadian clock progression in human cancer.

*PeerJ, 6,* e4327 and following.

Sternberg, D.A., et al. (2013). The largest human cognitive performance dataset reveals insights into the effects of lifestyle factors and aging.

*Frontiers in Human Neuroscience, 7,* 292 and following.

Taheri, S., et al. (2004). Short sleep duration is associated with reduced leptin, elevated ghrelin, and increased body mass index.

*PLoS Medicine, 1*(3), e62 and following.

Taylor, B.J., et al. (2016). Bedtime variability and metabolic health in midlife women: The SWAN Sleep Study.

*Sleep, 39*(2), 457-465.

Thompson, C.L., et al. (2011). Short duration of sleep increases risk of colorectal adenoma.

*Cancer, 117*(4), 841-847.

Thompson, C.L., & Li, L. 2012. Association of sleep duration and breast cancer OncotypeDX recurrence score.

*Breast Cancer Research and Treatment, 134*(3), 1291-1295.

Vaughn, C.B., et al. (2018). Sleep and breast cancer in the Western New York Exposures and Breast Cancer (WEB) Study.

*Journal of Clinical Sleep Medicine, 14*(1), 81-86.

Verkasalo, P.K., et al. (2005). Sleep duration and breast cancer: A prospective cohort study.

*Cancer Research, 65*(20), 9590-9600.

Viswanathan, A.N., et al, (2007). Night shift work and the risk of endometrial cancer.

*Cancer Research, 67*(21), 10618-10622.

White, A.J., et al. (2017). Sleep characteristics, light at night and breast cancer risk in a prospective cohort.

*International Journal of Cancer, 141*(11), 2204-2214.

Wu, A.H., et al. (2008). Sleep duration, melatonin and breast cancer among Chinese women in Singapore.

*Carcinogenesis, 29*(6), 1244-1248.

Zhao, H., et al. (2013). Sleep duration and cancer risk: A systematic review and meta-analysis of prospective studies.

*Asian Pacific Journal of Cancer Prevention, 14*(12), 7509-7515.

Alpha-Tocopherol, Beta Carotene Cancer Prevention Study Group. (1994). The effect of vitamin E and beta carotene on the incidence of lung cancer and other cancers in male smokers.

*The New England Journal of Medicine, 330*(15), 1029-1035.

# Chapter Twenty-Four

# Why Eating Meat From Mammals is Unhealthy for You

★ ★ ★

We have known for over half a century that those who consume large amounts of red meat (really, mammalian meat, such as beef, lamb, pork, venison, and other mammals – as well as their milk and dairy products) have heightened risks for cardiovascular diseases, cancers, diabetes, asthma, some kinds of arthritis, and autoimmune diseases. On the other hand, the human consumption of proteins from plants, does <u>not</u> correlate with these diseases.

Over 15 years ago, Professor Ajit Varki (University of California at San Diego) discovered that humans – unlike other mammals – do not produce Neu5Gc (N-glycolyl neuraminic acid). Instead, humans produce a one-molecule modification of Neu5Gc called Neu5Ac (Nacetyl neuraminic acid). **Dr. Varki's theory is that the consumption of Neu5Gc by humans turns on their immune systems to fight the ingested Neu5Gc molecules as if they were** invading germs. This process can (inappropriately) turn on their immune systems to fight themselves, and thereby produce <u>chronic inflammation</u>, which, in turn, can produce heart attacks, cancers, strokes, and other disease processes.

In humans, Neu5Gc is found in very high concentrations in tumors, and in even higher concentrations in tumors that have metastasized.

This phenomenon also explains why humans are the only mammal (indeed, the only animal) susceptible to malaria. To infect an animal, the plasmodia (malaria) parasite must first latch onto Neu5Ac on the surfaces of cells in order to gain entry into those cells, and only humans have that molecule on the surfaces of their cells.

There are real dangers when one eats egg yolks and mammalian meat. I strongly recommend not eating egg yolks, mammalian meat in general, and processed meats. These foods have high amounts of choline and lecithin, which the bacteria in the human gut convert to TMA (trimethylamine). Once absorbed into the blood stream, TMA is carried to the liver, where it is converted into TMAO (trimethylamineoxide), which causes a reduction in the good, healthy bacteria in the gut; this permits unhealthy bacteria to flourish. These events in the human body greatly increase the odds of a variety of dangerous conditions to develop, including **<u>heart attacks, strokes, cancers, and early death</u>**! (Zhong et al., 2019; Zheng, et al. 2019; Zhu, et al, 2016; Schiattarella, et al, 2017; Zhu, et al., 2017; Wang, et al., 2015; Wang, et al., 2011; Gregory, et al., 2015.)

**Recently published data also suggest that, at least in part, this**

**negative effect of consuming mammalian meat may be mediated via an effect on gut microbiota** (Kostik, et al, 2013; Shurney & Pauly, 2018; Shurney, 2019; Shivali, 2017; De Almeida, et al., 2019; Nogacka, et al., 2019).

<u>**Note**</u>**:** These cited references are based on people who regularly eat mammalian meat. In addition, recently published evidence (Alshahrani, et al., 2019) shows that **<u>even occasionally eating mammalian meat</u>** is likely to be <u>harmful to your body</u>.

# References

Alshahrani, S.M., et al. (2019). Red and processed meat and mortality in a low meat intake population.

*Nutrients, 11*(3), 622 and following.

De Almeida, C.V., et al. (2019). Role of diet and gut microbiota on colorectal cancer immunomodulation.

*World Journal of Gastroenterology, 5*(2), 151-162.

Hedlund, M., Padler-Karavani, V., Varki, N.M., & Varki, A. (2008). Evidence for a human-specific mechanism for diet and antibody-mediated inflammation in carcinoma progression.

*Proceedings of the National Academy of Sciences, 105*(48), 1893618941.

Kostic, A.D., et al. (2013). Fusobacterium nucleatum potentiates intestinal tumorigenesis and modulates the tumor-immune microenvironment.

*Cell Host & Microbe, 14*(2), 207-215.

Nogacka, A.M., et al. (2019). Xenobiotics formed during food processing: Their relation with the intestinal microbiota and colorectal cancer.

*International Journal of Molecular Science, 20*(8), 2051 and following.

Samrag, A.N., Pearce O.M.T., Läubli, H., Crittenden, A.N., Bergfeld, A.K., Banda, K., Gregg, C.J., Bingman, A.E., Secrest ,P., Diaz, S.L., Varki, N.M., & Varki, A. (2015). A red meat-derived glycan promotes inflammation and cancer progression.

*Proceedings of the National Academy of Sciences, 112*(2), 542-547.

Shah, S.C., et al. (2018). Microbial-host interactions in inflammatory bowel disease, functional bowel disease, obesity and obesity-related metabolic diseases.

*Gastroenterology, 155*(5), 1283-1286.

Shivali, S. (2017). We are not alone: A case for the human microbiome in extra intestinal diseases.

*Gut Pathogens, 9,* 13 and following.

Shurney, D. (2019). The gut microbiome: Unleashing the doctor within.

*American Journal of Lifestyle Medicine, 13*(3), 265-268.

Shurney, D., & Pauly, K. (2019). The gut microbiome and food as medicine: Healthy microbiomes = healthy humans.

*American Journal of Health Promotion, 33*(5), 821-824.

Tangvoranuntakul, P., Gagneux, P., Diaz, S., Bardor, M., Varki,

N., Varki, A., & Muchmore, E. (2003). Human uptake and incorporation of an immunogenic nonhuman dietary sialic acid.

*Proceedings of the National Academy of Sciences, 100*(21), 12045-12050.

[<u>Note</u>: **This study shows that consuming red meat increases the risk for cancers, etc.]**

# Chapter Twenty-Five

# Why Not Eating Enough Fruits, Vegetables, and Nuts/Seeds, and Too Much Sugar and Sugar Equivalents, is Always Unhealthy

———————— ★ ★ ★ ————————

ALL plants have anti-cancer chemicals in their cells – such chemicals protecting those plants from infections by bacteria, viruses, fungi, parasites, etc. that can cause cancer and other problems in those plants; and these chemicals grant similar protection to humans when they eat those plants. However, some plants have more robust protective systems than others. – A good example of a relatively nutritionally deficient food is iceberg lettuce.

Some data (Lv, et al., 2015) appears to show that spicy foods offer protection from cancers.

Another publication (Bressan & Kramer, 2016) cites 131 references that, collectively, support the authors' conclusions that **eating products that are made of flour, as well as dairy products (as** well as products made from corn and rice) greatly increases a person's risks for such diseases as schizophrenia, autism spectrum disorders, dementia, psychosis, bipolar disorder, depression, anxiety, postpartum psychosis, anorexia, celiac disease, fatigue, "foggy mind," arthritis, asthma, type 1 diabetes, eczema, and multiple sclerosis.

In addition to the effects of high rises in blood glucose from consuming food made from flour, another nutritional area of concern is glutens, including their stimulation of the release of opioid-like compounds (including zonulin) in the human body. The end effect appears to be a leaky gut (and possibly an overly porous blood-brain barrier, too), in which glutens and their breakdown products leak from a person's gut into their blood, and inappropriately activate a person's immune system which results in celiac disease (McGrann, 2019).

Furthermore, when a person's immune system is inappropriately activated (that is, over-activated), the risk for cancer goes up; however, the above-stated unhealthy negative effects of glutens can occur without symptoms. Therefore, I strongly recommend that you aim for a gluten-free life.

Note: To be gluten free you must avoid foods made of wheat (including its various varieties, such as kamut, spelt, triticale, and faro), rye, and barley.

Another study (Lassale, et al., 2018) cites abundant data that shows that, on average, those who have the best nutrition are the happiest! Thus, we can turn this concept in the opposite direction, and conclude that **less than stellar nutrition can contribute to your mental health being less than perfect**, and potentially to your having a less than totally bright outlook on life!

Finally, when you consume too much sugar and too much of what I call "sugar equivalents" (which refers to foods that become sugar by the time that they reach your stomach – such as all foods made of flour, including so-called "whole grain" flours), those sugars attach to cell membranes and proteins. On cell membranes, those sugar are converted to sorbitol. **When too many sorbitol molecules become attached to your cell membranes, the cells are killed.**

This destruction of cells can affect any cell in your body! For example, you can experience such effects as loss of taste, loss of smell, loss of hair, sexual disfunction, gangrene (requiring emergency amputation of the affected area), loss of eyesight (for example, retinal detachments and macular degeneration), some types of arthritis, type 2 diabetes, etc. Also, realize that following a "sugar heavy life" will promote plaque in your arteries, which will increase your risk not only for heart attacks and strokes, but also for many of the most common cancers and Alzheimer's!

**When you see balding or thinning hair in men and women, most of the time (probably 99% of the time!) it is due to a diet full of sugary foods and foods that are sugar equivalents; major food culprits are soft drinks, cold cereals, bread, pasta, crackers, pretzels, pastries, etc. High sugar diets destroy the follicles that produce hair! And do not allow yourself to be fooled into**

believing that "diet" sodas are any healthier – the <u>artificial sweeteners</u> are very unhealthy!

Other publications also support the above conclusions (Ondera, Nam, & Bissell, 2014; Graham, et al., 2012; Lin, et al., 2015; Fridlender, et al., 2015; O'Keef, et al., 2015; Boeing, et al., 2012).

The <u>bottom line</u>: **<u>You owe it to your body, your psyche, and your spiritual side to live as healthfully as possible</u>!** Also, remember that <u>you are only as healthy as your weakest link</u> (see Chapter 16).

# References

Boeing, H., et al. (2012). Critical review: Vegetables and fruit in the prevention of chronic diseases.

*European Journal of Nutrition, 51*(6), 637-663.

Bressan, P., & Kramer, P. (2016). Bread and other edible agents of mental disease.

*Frontiers in Human Neuroscience, 10,* 130 and following.

Fridlender, M., et al. (2015). Plant derived substances with anticancer activity: From folklore to practice.

*Frontiers in Plant Science, 6,* 799 and following.

Graham, N.A., et al. (2012). Glucose deprivation activates a metabolic and signaling amplification loop leading to cell death.

*Molecular Systems Biology, 8,* 589 and following.

Lassale, C., et al. (2018). Healthy dietary indices and risk of depressive outcomes: A systematic review and meta-analysis of observational studies.

*Molecular Psychiatry, 5,* 1 and following.

Lin, P.H., et al. (2015). Nutrition, dietary interventions and prostate cancer: The latest evidence.

*BMC Medicine, 13,* 3 and following.

Lv, J., et al. (2015). Consumption of spicy foods and total and cause specific mortality: Population based cohort study.

*British Medical Journal, 351,* h3942 and following.

McGrann, D. (2019). *The Accidental Cure.* Columbia, MD: Imagination Press, LLC.

Myerhardt, J.A., et al. (2012). Glycemic load and cancer recurrence and survival in patients with stage III colon cancer: Findings from CALGB 89803.

*Journal of the National Cancer Institute,104*(22), 1702-1711.

O'Keefe, S.J., et al. (2015). Fat, fiber and cancer risk in African Americans and rural Africans.

*Nature Communications, 6,* 6342 and following.

Onodera, Y., J-M Nan, J-M., & Bissell, M.J. (2014). Increased sugar uptake promotes oncogenesis via EPAC/RAP1 and O-GlcNAc pathways.

*The Journal of Clinical Investigation, 124*(1), 367-384.

# Chapter Twenty-Six

# The Truth About Multi-Vitamins and Supplements

――――――― ★ ★ ★ ―――――――

Many are fearful that they are deficient in their intake of vitamins and minerals, so they take "the easy way out" by taking **multi-vitamin pills and other supplements.** Sometimes physicians prescribe them for their patients; such prescribing physicians also prescribe them on their syndicated TV shows, and, in addition, claim to have knowledgeable, well-trained employees who verify scientific data to back up each of their claims that taking such supplements will improve your health. Well, guess what! If these physicians took the time to become familiar with the scientific literature in this area, they would realize that <u>**imperfect nutrition, plus vitamin pills and other supplements still equals imperfect nutrition!!!**</u>

The **three major possible exceptions** are **Vitamin D3, Vitamin B12** for vegan vegetarians, and for older individuals, and **iron for**

**pregnant women!** In addition, for persons on life support or who are frail and near the end of their lives, vitamin and mineral supplements may add a month or so of additional life. However, generally, <u>**you should only take vitamin and mineral supplements if there is a particularly good reason that is based on chemical testing**</u>**; the references listed below show that doing otherwise may increase your risk for cancer and other serious medical conditions!**

Just follow the prescriptions in this book to be certain that you get all the nutrients that your body needs – and by only eating foods that are both healthy and tasty!

**Those over 50 or so sometimes will have guts that no longer can effectively absorb Vitamin B-12. For them, they should use "<u>fast dissolving</u>" <u>Vitamin B-12</u> for sublingual (under the tongue) use.**

CANCER

# Note On African Americans and Other Persons of Color

Years ago, I learned of a disturbing report about what many African American mothers in the South were doing to their young children. When they pushed their children around their neighborhoods, they made sure that their children were shielded from direct sunlight because "they wanted their children to be lighter-skinned."

The horrible, unintended consequence is that their babies became <u>osteoporotic</u>, which manifested in their babies growing up bowlegged. Not enough sunlight reached these children to help their bodies produce **Vitamin D!** **Melanin** in the skin of these children also contributed to reducing the amount of ultraviolet rays from the sun going into their bodies to help produce strong, healthy bones!

Every cell in the human body has receptors for Vitamin D; these receptors bind to the Vitamin D molecules and "usher them into the cells," where they do their jobs of **<u>enhancing immune system function,</u>** building sex hormones (for example, estrogen and testosterone), building other hormones (for example, aldosterone), etc. **The fact that all cells have receptors for Vitamin D underscores the supreme importance of Vitamin D for <u>optimum health</u>**! Most physicians recommend that their patients <u>take **a Vitamin D pill (1,000 International Units)**</u> every day.

# References

Albanes, D., et al. (1996). Alpha-tocopherol and beta-carotene supplements and lung cancer incidence in the alpha-tocopherol, beta-carotene cancer prevention study: Effects of base-line characteristics and study compliance.

*Journal of the National Cancer Institute, 88*(21), 1560-1570.

Bjelakovic, G., et al. (2012). Antioxidant supplements for prevention of mortality in healthy participants and patients with various diseases.

*Cochrane Database Systematic Reviews, 3,* CD007176.

Bjelakovic, G., et al. (2007). Mortality in randomized trials of antioxidant supplements for primary and secondary prevention:

Review and meta-analysis.

*Journal of the American Medical Association, 297*(8), 842-857.

Bjelakovic, G., et al. (2004). Antioxidant supplements for prevention of gastrointestinal cancers: A systematic review and meta-analysis. *Lancet, 364*(9441), 1219-1228.

Hercberg, S., et al. (2007). Antioxidant supplementation increases the risk of skin cancers in women but not in men.

*Journal of Nutrition, 137*(9), 2098-2105.

Klein, E.A., et al. (2011). Vitamin E and the risk of prostate cancer: The Selenium and Vitamin E Cancer Prevention Trial (SELECT).

*Journal of the American Medical Association, 306*(14), 1549-1556.

Lonn, E., et al. (2005). Effects of long-term vitamin E supplementation on cardiovascular events and cancer: A randomized controlled trial.

*Journal of the American Medical Association, 293*(11), 1338-1347.

Mursu, J., et al. (2011). Dietary supplements and mortality rate in older women: The Iowa Women's Health Study.

*Archives of Internal Medicine, 171*(18), 1625-1633.

Neuhouser, M.L., et al. (2009). Multivitamin use and risk of cancer and cardiovascular disease in the Women's Health Initiative cohorts.

*Archives of Internal Medicine, 169*(3), 294-304.

Rautiainen, S., et al. (2016). Multivitamin use and the risk of hypertension in a prospective cohort study of women.

*Journal of Hypertension, 34*(8), 1513-1519.

Rautiainen, S., et al. (2015). Multivitamin use and cardiovascular disease in a prospective study of women.

*American Journal of Clinical Nutrition, 101*(1), 144-152.

Sesso, H.D., et al. (2012). Multivitamins in the prevention of cardiovascular disease in men: The Physicians' Health Study II randomized controlled trial.

*Journal of the American Medical Association, 308*(17), 1751-1760.

Sesso, H.D., et al. (2008). Vitamins E and C in the prevention of cardiovascular disease in men: The Physicians' Health Study II randomized controlled trial.

*Journal of the American Medical Association, 300*(18), 2123-2133.

Watson, J. (2013). Oxidants, antioxidants and the current incurability of metastatic cancers.

*Open Biology, 3*(1), 120144 and following.

**[NOTE: This author is James D Watson, who won a Nobel Prize with Francis Crick for determining the alpha helical structure of DNA.]**

[No authors listed]. (1994). The effect of vitamin E and beta carotene on the incidence of lung cancer and other cancers in male smokers. The Alpha-Tocopherol, Beta Carotene Cancer Prevention Study Group.

*The New England Journal of Medicine, 330*(15), 1029-1035.

# SECTION III

## The MORE: If You Desire to Delve Deeper into the Science

# Chapter Twenty- Seven

# How Applying EPIGENETICS Can Reduce Your Risk for Cancer

---  ★ ★ ★  ---

Epigenetics is the science of how you may control whether certain genes in the nuclei of the cells in your body are activated and/or deactivated to either make you <u>healthier</u> by reducing your risk for cancers (and many other medical conditions) when you make <u>healthy lifestyle choices</u>, or <u>unhealthier</u> when you make <u>unhealthy lifestyle choices</u>. However, realize that you cannot be healthier than your weakest health link. (See Chapter 16 for more on the weakest link concept.)

In the public realm, the field of epigenetics got its start from the seminal study of Dr. Dean Ornish and his research team (Ornish, et al., 2008). It is worth taking a look at this study to see how you can apply its lessons to improve your health.

Thirty men, with an average age of 62 years, and who were "low risk" for aggressive forms of prostate cancer (the men had a nonaggressive kind of prostate cancer), were enrolled in this study. At the beginning, needle prostate biopsies were taken to obtain baseline data, and other parameters were measured, including blood pressure, PSA (prostate specific antigen), free PSA, body weight and height, Body Mass Index (BMI – calculated from the person's height and weight), lipid profile, C-reactive protein, waist circumference, prostate volume, quality of life test, mental health test, psychological distress test, a SHOC2 array of gene expression measurements, and 406 transcripts (genome elements) – 18 of which had been activated and 388 of which had been deactivated by the end of the three-month <u>healthy-living experimental protocol</u>.

Over the three consecutive months, the "healthy-living protocol" was strictly followed, consisting of

- Low-fat (10% or less of caloric intake from fat), whole-foods, plant-based nutrition – supplemented with tofu, fish oil, vitamin E, and selenium
- Stress management techniques (practiced 60 minutes per day): Gentle yoga-based stretching, breathing, meditation, imagery, and progressive relaxation
- "Moderate" exercise (walking 30 minutes per day for 6 hours per week), and
- Participation in a psychosocial group (a one-hour support group session per week).

The key finding of this three-month diet/exercise/stress reduction protocol was **<u>a reduction in the level of active cancer-causing genes</u>**

<u>in the prostate</u> biopsy samples.

It is important to realize that some of the elements of this study protocol are now known to be ineffective – in particular, the vitamin/mineral supplements used in this study do not improve health. Also, higher levels of exercise (such as interval training for cardio conditioning, and demanding strength-building exercise) will improve health much more than the moderate-to-low level of walking prescribed in this study.

As a real-life hypothetical, consider Angelina Jolie's double mastectomy that she had after she discovered that her genetics included two known breast cancer-causing genes: <u>BRCA1</u> and <u>BRCA2</u>. Had she been my client, **I would have had a conversation with her to see if she were willing to lead a super-healthy lifestyle with respect to nutrition, sleep, strength-building exercise, cardio exercise, stress reduction, etc.** If she were willing to make major changes in <u>all</u> of these areas (if she happened to be deficient in any of them), I would have schooled her in all of the relevant specifics. Also, I would have noted that the newest technologies in imaging have made it possible to detect breast cancers much earlier than in the past, so she could put off considering the radical mastectomy surgery to see if her new, super healthy lifestyle succeeded in activating healthy genes and inactivating unhealthy genes.

Despite the above-described weaknesses, **a variety of confirming studies have been published since Ornish's 2008 publication – that is, studies that confirm that <u>your lifestyle choices can and do influence the expression of your genes</u>!** Specifically, many subsequent studies have shown that your healthy choices activate healthy genes, and your unhealthy choices activate unhealthy genes! (By the way, you should understand that all of the risk factors for cancer are also risk factors for heart attacks, strokes, high blood pressure, type 2 diabetes, dementia, and Alzheimer's disease!)

In addition, **see the section below in this chapter about the earlier discoveries of Dr. Bruce H. Lipton** (Lipton, 2016; Lipton, 2005/2006).

The references below present a selection of just <u>some</u> of the confirming epigenetic studies that have been published since 2008. You will readily appreciate the relevance of these studies when you read their titles. Basically, they corroborate the general discovery of Dr. Ornish that you can be rewarded for living a maximally healthy lifestyle (at least to the extent of current scientific knowledge, which can change in a heartbeat with future discoveries)! Many other references could have been listed, but just the titles of these references will give you a taste of the state-of-the-art research by scientists who study epigenetics. If you are a research scientist just starting to become knowledgeable about epigenetics, this list will serve you well as a starting point.

**Yet another aspect that has come to the fore in recent years is the role of lifestyle choices on your <u>gut microbiota</u> (Sivan, et al., 2015; Viaud, et al., 2014); these studies show that the kinds of bacteria in your gut respond to your nutritional and other choices, and <u>are critical to living a healthy life</u>! Furthermore, as but two examples (among many), chronic fatigue syndrome [also known as**

myalgic encephalomyeletes ("ME")] and rheumatoid arthritis appear to be caused by <u>unhealthy gut flora</u> (Griffin & Huffman, 2018; Lotan, et al., 2014; Maes, et al., 2013; Morris, et al., 2014; Shukla, et al., 2015; Lahiri, et al., 2014).

Also, **mitochondria in your cells (the "power houses" of your cells) work with your gut bacteria to decrease inflammation in your body, and to improve your endurance in endurance-requiring activities** (Clark & Mach, 2017; Hood, et al., 2011; Radak, et al., 2008).

Thus, **a range of studies** (Diab, et al., 2016; Gaudin, et al., 2008; Griffin & Huffman, 2019; Jafri, et al., 2016; Lotan, et al., 2014; Maes, et al., 2013; Morris, et al., 2014; Plasqui, 2008; Shukla, et al., 2015) **collectively show how the diverse components of your body work in concert to control and improve the many parts of your body! Also, Lahiri and coworkers** (Lahiri, et al., 2014) **reviewed the records of 25,455 people and found** <u>that those who smoked, were overweight, or had diabetes were more likely to develop rheumatoid arthritis, compared to "normal," non-arthritic people</u>!

Lifestyle choices that can <u>reduce symptoms of rheumatoid arthritis</u> and <u>reduce inflammation</u> include **exercise, nutrition, and reducing excess weight,** as is shown in a variety of studies (GarcíaPoma, 2007; Gaudin, et al., 2008; Hoström, et al., 2001; Lahiri, et al., 2014; Lee, et al., 2006; Lithell, et al., 1983; Marlow, et al., 2013; McKellar, et al., 2007; Müller, et al., 2001; Neuberger, et al., 2007; Plasqii, 2008; Shapiro, et al., 1996; Sköldstam, et al., 1979; Zhang, et al., 2014; Zhou & Sun, 2018).

Finally, Wang, et al. (Wang, et al., 2017) reviews studies on the effects of <u>vaccinations</u> on the risk of getting lupus and rheumatoid arthritis.

The lessons from Epigenetics are simple and straight-forward. **<u>YOU, and YOU ALONE, have the power to control your genetic destiny</u>**! Although spiritual leaders and other leaders have taught this for many millennia (though they knew nothing about anything called epigenetics), we now have consensus in the scientific community! Specifically, **we now know that you can deactivate unhealthy genes and activate healthy genes in your body simply through <u>healthy lifestyle choices</u>**!

Of course, we do not yet know all the nuances and capabilities of this phenomenon. **However, the findings to date greatly expand on previously discovered capabilities of your genetic system, including, for example, the <u>DNA repair mechanism</u> that periodically scours your DNA for damage (from sunlight-derived ultraviolet light, X-rays, gamma radiation, etc.; from the consumption of unhealthy nutrients; from an insufficient amount of exercise; etc.), and then makes the needed repairs (Gerard, et al., 2019)**. Another reference addresses the related area of telomere length relative to pancreatic cancer (Campa, et al., 2019).

So, as noted above, Dean Ornish and his lab showed **that <u>a 90-day change in diet and other lifestyle factors switched off the activities of over 500 genes</u>** – many of which were critical to the formation of tumors. However, scientists had been working a bit earlier on how the human body accomplished these epigenetic effects, as revealed in the early data of <u>Bruce H. Lipton</u> (Lipton,

2005/2006; Lipton, 2016). In addition, Lipton has posted lectures on this subject on YouTube.

**It is not within the scope of this chapter to delve deeply into the numerous details of Dr. Lipton's work; however, two real-life examples will suffice to show the massive power of his discoveries.**

**Example 1.** Lipton relates how, in 1952, a British physician tried to treat a 15-year-old boy's warts using hypnosis (Lipton, 2016, p. 117). Under hypnosis, the physician told him that he would cure his own leathery, grotesque skin that was on his arms, including warts. A week later, his physician met with him and was happy to note that the skin on his arms was back to normal; so, his physician took him to the surgeon who had referred the boy to him. The physician was surprised when the surgeon pointed out that he had made a mistake in his initial diagnosis. In fact, **the boy had an "<u>incurable condition</u>" called "congenital ichthyosis." Thus, the boy and his physician had accomplished something that was considered impossible!** – And the boy went on to live a normal life!

**Example 2.** Gardeners have found that planting basil near chili seeds produces spicy food. For example, the presence of basil enhanced the germination rates of chili seeds. Furthermore, they discovered that this occurred even when light, chemical, and physical touch (the three parameters typically studied by scientists for their effects on subjects) were blocked. Thus, **these researchers concluded that these three signaling mechanisms were "clearly not necessary for chili seeds and basil plants to sense each other's**

presence." Dr. Lipton (Lipton, 2016, pp. 110-111) **concluded that these results were the result of "<u>quantum energetic communication</u>."**

These two examples, and many others in the book, support not only the concept that <u>the mind</u> (i.e., <u>belief</u>) can not only <u>override gene expression</u>, but also that <u>other organisms</u> (plants, lower animals, and even single-celled organisms) <u>can communicate among themselves</u>; and that quantum mechanical mechanisms and principles provide the basis of these findings!

Thus, **if a person believes that they can cure their cancer on their own, and if they also follow the other biological principles of this book (nutrition, sleep, exercise, stress reduction, weight loss if needed, avoiding pollution and toxins, etc.), then their odds of success are significantly enhanced!**

Another way of looking at epigenetics is that, **now, in one fell swoop, you are able to make several quantum jumps-worth of power and capability that, heretofore, were unimaginable!** Just think! **You are even more powerful than you ever realized! And all that you must do to fully harness this power is**

## JUST ONE THING:

## LIVE A HEALTHY LIFE!!!

[A Modest Suggestion: Save yourself some time, energy, and aggravation, and use this book as <u>your roadmap</u>, or at least your starting point!]

# References

Ben-Shmuel, S., et al. (2016). Metabolic syndrome, type 2 diabetes, and cancer: Epidemiology and potential mechanisms.

*Handbook of Experimental Pharmacology, 233,* 355-372.

Campa, D., et al. (2019). Genetic determinants of telomere length and risk of pancreatic cancer: A PANDoRA study.

*International Journal of Cancer, 144*(6), 1275-1283.

Carr, P.R., et al. (2018). Healthy lifestyle factors associated with lower risk of colorectal cancer irrespective of genetic risk.

*Gastroenterology, 155*(6), 1805-1815.

Cheung, A.C., et al. (2017). Epigenetics in the primary biliary cholangitis and primary sclerosing cholangitis.

*Seminars in Liver Disease, 37*(2), 159-174.

Clark, A., & Mach, N. (2017). The crosstalk between the gut microbiota and mitochondria during exercise.

*Frontiers in Physiology, 8,* 319 and following.

Diab, M., et al. (2016). The role of microRNAs in the diagnosis and treatment of pancreatic adenocarcinoma.

*Journal of Clinical Medicine 5(6), 59 and following.*

Erben, V., et al. (2019). Strong associations of a healthy lifestyle with all stages of colorectal carcinogenesis: Results from a large cohort of participants of screening colonoscopy.

*International Journal of Cancer, 144(9), 2135-2143.*

García-Poma, A., et al. (2007). Obesity is independently associated with impaired quality of life in patients with rheumatoid arthritis.

*Clinical Rheumatology, 26(11), 1831-1835.*

Gaudin, P., et al. (2008). Is dynamic exercise beneficial in patients with rheumatoid arthritis?

*Joint, Bone, Spine: revue de rhumatisme, 75(1), 11-17.*

Gerard, E., et al. (2019). Familial breast cancer and DNA repair genes: Insights into known and novel susceptibility genes from the GENESIS study, and implications for multigene panel testing.

*International Journal of Cancer, 144(8), 1962-1974.*

Griffin, T.M., & Huffman, K.M. (2016). Editorial: Insulin resistance: Releasing the brakes on synovial inflammation and osteoarthritis?

*Arthritis & Rheumatology (Hoboken, NJ), 68(6), 1330-1333.*

Hood, D.A., et al. (2011). Mechanisms of exercise-induced

mitochondrial biogenesis in skeletal muscle: Implications for health and disease.

*Comprehensive Physiology, 1,* 1119-1134.

Hoström, I., et al. (2001). A vegan diet free of gluten improves the signs and symptoms of rheumatoid arthritis: The effects on arthritis correlate with a reduction in antibodies to food antigens.

*Rheumatology (Oxford, England), 40*(10), 1175-1179.

Jafri, M.A., et al. (2016). Roles of telomeres and telomerase in cancer, and advances in telomerase-targeted therapies.

*Genome Medicine, 8*(1), 69 and following.

Kanherkar, R.R., et al. (2017). Epigenetic mechanisms of integrative medicine.

*Evidence-Based Complementary and Alternative Medicine, 2017,* 43655429 and following.

Labbé, D.P., et al. (2015). Role of diet in prostate cancer: The epigenetic link.

*Oncogene, 34*(36), 4683-4691.

Lahiri, M., et al. (2014). Using lifestyle factors to identify individuals at higher risk of inflammatory polyarthritis (results from the European Prospective Investigation of Cancer-Norfolk and the Norfolk Arthritis Register - the EPIC-2-NOAR Study).

*Annals of the Rheumatic Diseases, 73*(1), 219-226.

Lee, E.O., et al. (2006). Effects of regular exercise on pain, fatigue, and disability in patients with rheumatoid arthritis.

*Family and Community Health, 29(4), 320-327.*

Lipton, B.H. (2005/2006). *The Biology of Belief – Unleashing the Power of Consciousness, Matter & Miracles.*

Lipton, B.H. (2016). *The Biology of Belief – Unleashing the Power of Consciousness, Matter & Miracles.*

Lithell, H., et al. (1983). A fasting and vegetarian diet treatment trial on chronic inflammatory disorders.

*Acta Dermato-Venereologica, 63(5), 397-403.*

Lotan, D., et al. (2014). Behavioral and neural effects of intrastriatal infusion of anti-streptococcal antibodies in rats.

*Brain, Behavior, and Immunity, 38, 249-262.*

Maes, M., et al. (2013). In myalgic encephalomyelitis/chronic fatigue syndrome, increased autoimmune activity against 5-HT is associated with immuno-inflammatory pathways and bacterial translocation.

*Journal of Affective Disorders, 150(2), 223-230.*

Marlow, G., et al. (2013). Transcriptomics to study the effects of a Mediterranean-inspired diet on inflammation in Crohn's disease patients.

*Human Genomics, 7(1), 24 and following*

McKellar, G., et al. (2007). A pilot study of a Mediterranean-type diet intervention in female patients with rheumatoid arthritis living in areas of social deprivation in Glasgow.

*Annals of the Rheumatic Diseases, 66*(9), 1239-1243.

Medvedeva, Y.A., et al. (2015). EpiFactors: A comprehensive database of human epigenetic factors and complexes.

*Database: The Journal of Biological Databases and Curation, 2015,* bav067 and following.

Morris, G., et al. (2014). The emerging role of autoimmunity in myalgic encephalomyelitis/chronic fatigue syndrome (ME/cfs).

*Molecular Neurobiology, 49*(2), 741-756.

Müller, H., et al. (2001). Fasting followed by vegetarian diet in patients with rheumatoid arthritis: A systematic review.

*Scandinavian Journal of Rheumatology, 30*(1), 1-10.

Neuberger, G.B., et al. (2007). Predictors of exercise and effects of exercise on symptoms, function, aerobic fitness, and disease outcomes of rheumatoid arthritis.

*Arthritis and Rheumatism, 57*(6), 943-952.

O'Keefe, S.J., et al. (2015). Fat, fibre and cancer risk in African Americans and rural Africans.

*Nature Communications, 6,* 6342 and following.

Ornish, D., et al. (2008). Changes in prostate gene expression in men undergoing an intensive nutrition and lifestyle intervention.

*Proceedings of the National Academy of Sciences, 105*(24), 8369-8374.

Plasquí, G. (2008). The role of physical activity in rheumatoid arthritis.

*Physiology and Behavior, 94*(2), 270-275.

Radak, Z., et al. (2008). Exercise, oxidative stress and hormesis.

*Ageing Research Reviews, 7,* 34-42.

Shapiro, J.A., et al. (1996). Diet and rheumatoid arthritis in women: A possible protective effect of fish consumption.

*Epidemiology, 7*(3), 256-263.

Shukla, S.K., et al. (2015). Changes in gut and plasma microbiome following exercise challenge in myalgic encephalomyelitis/chronic fatigue syndrome (ME/CFS).

*PLoS One, 10*(12), e145453 and following.

Sivan, A., et al. (2015). Commensal Bifidobacterium promotes antitumor immunity and facilitates anti-PD-L1 efficacy.

*Science, 350*(6264), 1084-1090.

Sköldstam, L., et al. (1979). Effect of fasting and lactovegetarian diet on rheumatoid arthritis.

*Scandinavian Journal of Rheumatology, 8*(4), 249-255.

Slattery, M.L., et al. (2015). Differential gene expression in colon tissue associated with diet, lifestyle, and related oxidative stress.

*PLoS One, 10*(7), e0134406 and following.

Song, M., et al. (2018). Fiber intake and survival after colorectal cancer diagnosis.

*JAMA Oncology, 4*(1), 71 and following.

Tabung, F.K., et al. (2018). Association of dietary inflammatory potential with colorectal cancer risk in men and women.

*JAMA Oncology, 4*(3), 366-373.

Theodoratou, E., et al. (2017). Nature, nurture and cancer risks: Genetic and nutritional contributions to cancer.

*Annual Review of Nutrition, 37*, 293-320.

Van Praet, L., et al. (2013). Microscopic gut inflammation in axial spondyloarthritis: A multiparametric predictive model.

*Annals of the Rheumatic Diseases, 72*(3), 414-417.

Viaud, S., et al. (2014). Why should we need the gut microbiota to respond to cancer therapies?

*Oncoimmunology, 3*(1), e27574 and following.

Wang, B., et al. (2017). Vaccinations and risk of systemic lupus erythematosus: A systematic review and meta-analysis.

*Autoimmunity Reviews, 16*(7), 756-765.

Zhang, J.X., et al. (2014). Associations between P TPN2

polymorphisms and susceptibility to ulcerative colitis and Crohn's disease: A meta-analysis.

*Inflammation Research, 63*(1), 71-79.

Zhou, Y., & Sun, M. (2018). A meta-analysis of the relationship between body mass index and risk of rheumatic arthritis.

*EXCLI Journal, 17,* 1079-1089.

# Chapter Twenty- Eight

# Innovations in Cancer Research

* ★ *

A number of innovations in cancer research have resulted since the genome project in Rockville, Maryland was completed – in which the entire human genome was determined! Perhaps the greatest innovation is the ability to now focus on the individual's needs – based strictly on their unique genes, instead of a one-size-fits-all approach. Furthermore, doctors and geneticists can now collaborate to bring the best possible treatment for each cancer patient!

Below, a number of cancer treatments are listed – some based on gene therapy, and others requiring drugs or surgery. Perhaps the best attack against many forms of cancers is to **build <u>the healthiest immune system possible</u>** in each patient since, every day, everyone has millions of "mini-cancers" that are looking for toe holds from which to grow into malignant cancers!

Listed below are a few innovations that are used in current cancer research.

**Genome Sequencing**: This technique allows researchers to read and decipher the genetic information (that is, the sequence of the individual DNA molecules) of anything from bacteria to plants to animals.

The first genome sequencing study was published by Sjoblom et al., 2006 on human breast and colorectal tumors.

The advantages of genome sequencing are numerous. First, with the advent of the Cancer Genome Project, oncologists and geneticists are now able to identify driver genes, which are the principal genes that are responsible for causing a particular cancer. Second, by gathering a large amount of data on such aberrant genes, the cost of cancer treatments will be driven down. Third, genome sequencing, an example of "precision medicine," now aids in prescribing a recommendation based on information specifically designed for each individual patient. For example, all breast cancers do not respond the same way to a given treatment. As a result of recent advances in cancer research, we are now better understanding the role that genetics plays in contracting a cancer, as well as in treating a cancer.

**Immunotherapy** is a therapy that is based on the concept that **a super healthy immune system will allow a patient's own body to effectively fight off a cancer!**

The National Cancer Institute website outlines a number of immunotherapy treatment options:

1. **Immune checkpoint inhibitors** are drugs that help a patient's immune system by establishing various biochemical checkpoints in their body. These checkpoints are amenable to the action of certain drugs that keep the patient's immune system from causing whole-body inflammation. As a result, these biochemical checkpoints allow the patient's immune system to respond better to certain anti-cancer treatments.

2. **T-cell transfer therapy** is a treatment that boosts the natural ability of a person's own T cells to fight cancer. These cells, which are taken directly from a cancer patient's tumor, are placed in a petri dish, where they multiply so that a more robust response can be mounted against the patient's cancer when they are infused intravenously back into the patient.

3. **Monoclonal antibodies** are proteins that are designed and created in a lab to boost the level of function of the patient's immune system. These monoclonal antibodies function just like (and act in concert, to increase the level of function of) the patient's regular antibodies to search out and destroy cancer cells in the patient's body.

**Surgery:** One way to treat cancer is by the "traditional" procedure of cutting the cancer out of the patient's body. Generally, this surgery can be painful and often is costly.

However, less invasive technological improvements have been made, such as **laser surgery,** in which a laser beam is directed at a tumor to destroy most or all of the cancer – with minimum damage to adjacent tissues.

**Cryosurgery,** also a relatively new technology, uses very cold liquid nitrogen or liquid argon to eradicate cancer by more or less selective freezing. This type of surgery is often used in early stages of growth for cancers of the skin and the cervix, as well as other cancers.

Other types of surgeries include <u>minimally invasive surgery</u> and <u>open surgery</u>.

Minimally invasive surgery usually accesses a cancer by small cuts made in the patient's skin. A laparoscope (a long thin tube with a camera) is a tool that often is used to image the location of a tumor so that small surgical tools can then remove the cancer.

In open surgery (think of this as "traditional" surgery), cuts are made in the patient's body to remove a tumor – sometimes including removing cancerous lymph nodes.

**Radiation Therapy/Radiotherapy** is a treatment that uses high doses of radiation to kill or shrink cancers. This type of therapy is expensive because it requires treatment by specialist health practitioners, and the radiation-producing machines are expensive. Also, there is a large risk with radiation therapy because the patient's body cannot safely withstand continued high doses of radiation – especially because <u>the radiation also damages nearby (non-cancerous) tissues</u>. Hence, if a patient receives radiation in one area of their body, there must be careful consideration when considering the possibility of needing subsequent doses of radiation – including the probable negative impact on healthy, non-cancerous tissues.

There are <u>two general types of radiation therapy</u> that are used to treat cancers. For **internal radiation therapy,** a liquid or solid piece of radioactive material is placed in or near the cancer cells. This process, also called **brachytherapy,** utilizes seeds, ribbons, or capsules that contain a radioactive material. This type of therapy is often used when thyroid glands need to be removed in order for the patient to switch to Synthroid (synthetic thyroid hormone). Open surgery cannot reach all of the small traces of thyroid tissue that form two "trails" of thyroid tissue that are in the chest as a result of embryological movement as a fetus develops into a young child, and then into an adult. In this case, all the thyroid tissue in the patient is irradiated with radioactive iodine that is administered intravenously into the patient. The radioactive iodine it taken up only into thyroid tissue. Also, the radioactive iodine has a "short half-life," which means that it remains radioactive only a very short time, which greatly reduces the possible negative effects of getting too much radiation exposure.

<u>**Chemotherapy**</u> is a cancer treatment that kills cancer through the use of drugs. Whenever we talk about "traditional" cancer treatment, chemotherapy (using methotrexate) is the treatment that is referred to. Chemotherapy works by shrinking and killing the cancers.

Traditional chemotherapy typically has many strong effects – including not only killing cancer cells, but <u>also killing healthy cells</u>! Patients who undergo traditional chemotherapy usually feel incredibly tired, and also experience other effects, such as extreme nausea. All of these effects combine to make the treatment so horrific that these patients claim that they would never undergo chemotherapy again if their cancer returned!

**Chemotherapy can be administered in several ways:**

- **Oral**

    The chemotherapeutic medication comes in pills, capsules, or liquids that are swallowed

- **Intravenous (IV)**

    The chemotherapeutic medication is administered directly into a vein

- **Injection**

    The chemotherapeutic medication is administered by a shot into a muscle in the arm, thigh, or hip, or under the skin in a fatty part of the arm, leg, or belly

- **Intrathecal**

    The chemotherapeutic medication is injected into the space between the layers of tissue that cover the brain and spinal cord (technically, injected under the arachnoid membrane)

- **Intraperitoneal (IP)**

    The chemotherapeutic medication is administered directly by syringe and needle into the peritoneal cavity – the area in a body that contains organs, such as intestines, stomach, and liver

- **Intra-arterial (IA)**

    The chemotherapeutic medication is injected directly into the <u>artery</u> that leads to the cancer

- **Topical**

    The chemotherapeutic medication comes in a cream that is rubbed onto the skin

Chemotherapy is also expensive due to **<u>Stem Cell Research</u>:** In this area of research and practice, blood-forming stem cells are used to produce new blood cells. Essentially, a patient receives an injection of these blood-forming stem cells that replenish the patient's low, unhealthy levels of blood cells. These stem cells can come from the patient, from a twin or a relative, or from another donor.

# Reference

Sjoblom, T., et al. (2006). The consensus coding sequences of human breast and colorectal cancers.

*Science. 314 (5797), 268–274.*

## Chapter Twenty-Nine

## The Relentless Flood of Scientific Articles on Cancer

---⋆ ★ ⋆---

An astounding, mind-bending statistic about cancer research **publications** was recently reported by a TV station's news broadcast:

> **On average, over 6,000 cancer studies are published every month!**

The human mind cannot assimilate this much information, so researchers have dumped these studies and their conclusions into a single large database.

Medical doctors who treat patients who are not responding well to conventional treatments for cancer cleverly search this information, and often are able to direct their patients' bodies into cancer remission with new methodologies! Virtually every major

# CANCER

cancer treatment program in the United States and elsewhere has ventured into this new, uncharted territory.

Cancer research scientists also smartly mine this database for nuggets of knowledge that will expand their research horizons.

Thus, this is a benefit to living in THE INFORMATION AGE! Or, as some prefer, this is living in THE DIGITAL AGE.

# Chapter Thirty

# Complications Relating to Cancer

★ ★ ★

If you seek more knowledge relating to the possible changes and complications that scientists encounter in cancer research, check out the following references; collectively, these references address complications that can arise from cancer – such as **metastasizing to other tissues and organs.** This is **the greatest general concern,** because when the cancer stays within the one tissue or organ, it is not nearly as dangerous as when it spreads elsewhere. For example, when female breast cancer stays within the breast, it usually is not as dangerous as when it spreads to the brain!

The Fasano reference addresses **the roles of your gut bacteria and your gut health** to reduce your odds of getting cancer. The most important point of this reference is that you need to take care of your gut bacteria in order to be healthy! That is, **what is good for your gut bacteria is good for your overall health**! Thus, all of your lifestyle

# CANCER

choices come to bear here: exercise, sleep, stress reduction, maintaining a healthy body weight, etc. because **they all impact your gut bacteria!**

# References

Fasano, A. (2011). Zonulin and its regulation of intestinal barrier function: The biological door to inflammation, autoimmunity, and cancer.

*Physiological Reviews, 91*(1), 151-175.

Gati, A., et al. (2014). Obesity and renal cancer. Role of adipokines in the tumor-immune system conflict.

*Oncoimmunology 3,* e27810 and following.

Geijsen, A.J.M.R., et al. (January 21, 2019). Plasma metabolites associated with colorectal cancer: a discovery-replication strategy.

*International Journal of Cancer, ijc.32146* and following.

**[Note: These researchers identified 691 metabolic features that allowed them to discriminate between colorectal cancer patients and controls.]**

Gillen, J.B., et al. (2016). Twelve weeks of sprint interval training improves indices of cardiometabolic health similar to traditional endurance training despite a five-fold lower exercise volume and time commitment.

*PLos One 11*(4), e0154075 and following.

Lerman, B., et al. (2018). Oxytocin and cancer: An emerging link.

*World Journal of Clinical Oncology 9*(5), 74-82.

Weroha, S.J., & Haluska, P. (2012). The insulin-like growth factor system in cancer.

*Endocrinology & Metabolism Clinics of North America 41*(2), 335-350.

# SECTION IV

## CONCLUDING REMARKS AND PERSPECTIVES: Putting It All Together

# Chapter Thirty-One

# Total Health, Total Health, Total Health

★★★

*Either You Fully Embrace It, or You Won't
Reap the Benefits that You Seek!!!*

Undoubtedly, you have heard that the three most important things in real estate that determine the value of real property are **Location! Location! Location!**

In the health arena, now, due to the principles outlined in this book, **the three most important things to consider regarding your health are <u>Total Health! Total Health! Total Health!</u>**

**The reason this is true is that, if you do not fully embrace <u>TOTAL</u> Health, then you will fall victim to The Weakest Link concept,** as was discussed in Chapter 16. Recall that the example of smoking was discussed – with the conclusion that no amount of smoking is healthy, including inhaling second-hand smoke, or being subjected to third hand smoke. Thus, in general, **if (and when) you**

- consume sugary sodas and other unhealthy foods,
- fail to get enough of the right kind of exercise,
- fail to get a sufficient amount of deep sleep virtually every night, or
- allow your body to be overweight, sooner or later, <u>you should expect unhealthy results,</u> as discussed in the previous chapters. One of the problems in saying this is that you could already have unhealthy results – but not be aware of them – because **there may be ZERO discernible symptoms**! And you should **also expect to reap "the benefits" in the form of <u>an early demise</u>** – probably preceded by one or more cancers, cardiovascular diseases, Alzheimer's disease, and/or diabetes – to name a few!

Having said that, I believe that it is important to quell a common myth or mistaken belief. To address one specific example, the singer Kelly Clarkson has stated publicly that she was more comfortable at a higher weight, which obviously was unhealthy. The almost certain "fact" is that her body weight was at a higher set point. By far, the **best way that I know to <u>re-set your body weight set point</u> is to engage in regular, demanding exercise – especially Interval Training!** Of course, a modicum of strength-building exercise each week would also contribute substantially to weight loss success, as would healthy nutrition and plenty of deep sleep virtually every night.

The reason I use the verbiage "almost certain fact" is that I have not seen Kelly's health and medical records. For example, she could have had any of a variety of hormonal issues (thyroid, pituitary, adrenal, or other hormonal irregularities) or other medical issues that could have contributed to her being overweight. That is one reason why it is important to undergo a thorough medical exam prior to commencing a weight loss program! [Since then, it has been publicized that Kelly had a thyroid issue. Once it was corrected, her excess weight melted away without changes in her lifestyle choices, as far as we know.] However, since then, she has appears to have regained excess, unhealthy weight.

**A recent article (Shaw, 2019) addressed the role of <u>inflammation</u> in most – if not all – of the common chronic diseases, including the history of how inflammation became recognized for its causative participation in a multitude of physiological and biochemical processes (both positive and negative) in the human body!** Not surprisingly, <u>**inflammation**</u> **was identified as the starting point of most cancers, many types of arthritis, type 2 diabetes, plaques in arteries (think risks for heart attacks and strokes), etc.!**

A very important conclusion of one study is that "studies comparing the risks of migrants (particularly from Asia to the United States) to the risks of their offspring report **major increases in risks between first, second, and third generations, pointing to <u>changes in lifestyle and environmental exposure, rather than genetics</u>.**" (Ball, 2016; underlining for emphasis is by present author.) **Thus, a significant portion of deaths each year are due to <u>failure to apply simple,** *preventable* **actions</u>!**

Another study concluded that <u>an unhealthy diet causes more deaths world-wide than any other risk factor</u> (Afshin, et al., 2019)! The authors of this reference studied the roughly <u>11 million deaths</u> each year due to <u>nutritional deficiencies</u> from 1990 to 2017, including <u>data from 195 countries</u>.

Another study examined how the excess of light in the modern world can adversely affect mood (read also, mental health!) (Bedrosian, et al., 2013).

The Lee & Skerrett, reference concludes that **physical inactivity is responsible for increased deaths ("burden of disease") from coronary heart disease (6%), type 2 Diabetes(7%), breast cancer (10%), and colon cancer (10%)** (Lee & Skerrett, 2001).

**Other studies emphasize the extreme importance and effectiveness of lifestyle factors in preventing cancers** (Carr, et al., 2018; Erben, et al, 2019; Fasano, 2011; Theodoratou, 2017).

Thus, the prescriptions of this book and this chapter have rock solid foundations in the bio-medical literature!

# Reference

Afshin, A., et al. (2019). Health effects of dietary risks in 195 countries, 1990-2017: A systematic analysis for the Global Burden of Disease Study 2017.

*The Lancet, 393,* 791-846.

Ball, L.J., et al. (2016). The pathophysiologic role of disrupted circadian and neuroendocrine rhythms in breast carcinogenesis.

*Endocrine Reviews, 37*(5), 450-456.

Bedrosian, T.A., et al. (2013). Influence of the modern light environment on mood.

*Molecular Psychiatry, 18,* 751-757.

Carr, P.R., et al. (2018). Healthy lifestyle factors associated with lower risk of colorectal cancer irrespective of genetic risk.

*Gastroenterology, 155*(6), 1805-815.

Erben, V., et al. (2019). Strong associations of a healthy lifestyle with all stages of colorectal carcinogenesis: Results from a large cohort of participants of screening colonoscopy.

*International Journal of Cancer, 144*(9), 2135-2143.

Fasano, A. (2011). Zonulin and its regulation of intestinal barrier function: The biological door to inflammation, autoimmunity, and cancer.

*Physiological Reviews, 91*(1), 151-175.

Ford, C.T., et al. (2016). Identification of (poly)phenol treatments that modulate the release of pro-inflammatory cytokines by human lymphocytes.

*British Journal of Nutrition, 115*(10), 1699-1710.

Lee, I.M., & Skerrett, P.J. (2001). Physical activity and all-cause mortality: What is the dose-response relation?

*Medicine and Science in Sports and Exercise, 33*(6 Suppl), S459-S471.

Martinez-Valdes, E., et al. (2017). Differential motor unit changes after endurance or high-intensity interval training.

*Medicine and Science in Sports and Exercise 49*(6), 1126-1136.

Niemelä, M., et al. (2019). Intensity and temporal patterns of physical activity and cardiovascular disease risk in midlife.

*Preventive Medicine 124,* 33-41.

Shaw, J. (May-June, 2019). Raw and red-hot. Could inflammation be the cause of myriad chronic diseases?

*Harvard Magazine,* 46 and following.

Theodoratou, E., et al. (2017). Nature, nurture and cancer risks: Genetic and nutritional contributions to cancer.

*Annual Review of Nutrition, 37,* 293-320.

## Chapter Thirty-Two

## NO GUARANTEES!!!

———————— ✶ ✮ ✶ ————————

A person may be diagnosed with cancer even when they have led a close-to-exemplary lifestyle for decades.

Thus, the message is that we do not know about ALL of the possible causes of cancer, and how to fully prevent it. Think of it in statistical The more things you can check off in your anti-cancer lifestyle checklist, the more likely you are to prevent it; however, 100% success is not yet attainable.

However, you absolutely should do obvious things, such as: **have your basement checked for radioactive radon,** a long-known carcinogen.

Wean yourself off drinking water from plastic bottles because of the micro particles that linger in them (now known to be carcinogenic), and avoid plastic water bottles and other sources of plastic that have been produced using plastic hardeners [plasticizers, including BPA (see earlier chapter herein) and other usually unspecified plasticizers] – not only including for the linings of cans used for food, but also possibly for linings in metal bottles for carrying water and other beverages.

Fluoride in drinking water has allegedly been linked to cancer risks, according to social media and other sources. One study presents data that show that abortions can be caused by high levels of fluoride in drinking water (Moghaddam, et al., 2018); however, other studies show no linkage between fluoride levels in drinking water and cancer (Blakey, et al., 2014; Harrison, 2005; Tohyama, 1996; Whitford, 1992; Yang, et al., 2000). Nonetheless, if fluoride in drinking water can cause abortions (Moghaddam, 2018), that is a serious and troubling finding! Such data raise the obvious question as to whether other health risks remain to be identified!

**Other studies show how you can reap the rewards from adopting healthy lifestyle choices, and the unhealthy consequences when you do not** (Lindeberg, et al., 1994; Rarau, et al., 2017; Frostegård, et al., 2007!

Another area of concern is that of the possible effects of <u>dyes in printing inks</u> and other products – think of dyes in and on magazines and books and in clothing, etc., that could be absorbed from touching – including dyes on photocopies from a printer! (Studies relating to various dyes include Kulshreshtha, et al., 2011; Lucová, M., et al. (2013); Platzek, 2010; Wang, et al., 2005; Al-Saleh & Al-Enazi, 2011; and News Release, 2013). – But the obvious question is **how do you best protect yourself from such dyes?** Unfortunately, we need more data than is presently available! Should you be a hypochondriac and wash your hands every 5 minutes when you are handling such dye sources (for example, touching a photo in a magazine)? Or is 20 minutes, or 2 hours, a "reasonable compromise?" Personally, I tentatively aim for washing my hands about every 2 hours when my hands are in contact with dye sources (usually books, magazines, and photocopies); when new data are published, I will rethink this personal standard.

There is an important study that shows that you can have extremely negative effects on the genes in your cells when you consume even small quantities of alcohol (Harpaz, et al., 2015). See also Chapter 11 above.

Finally, I think it is wise to consider nutrition practices that have passed "the test of time" (for example, thousands of years!) in cultures in Africa, China, India, etc. A Chinese friend of mine incorporates many of the principles in this book in her nutrition. One of her concoctions comprises many kinds of beans, millet, sorghum, Chinese dates, walnuts, etc.

Another of her favorite recipes is a smoothie made from carrots and almonds, plus 1 tablespoon of black sesame powder and 1 tablespoon of black bean powder. She likes to consume this before lunch. She believes that this is responsible for changing her hair color from grey back to black. (<u>Note</u>: Black sesame seeds are much smaller than "conventional" sesame seeds; in addition, black sesame seeds are <u>much more nutritious</u> than our usual sesame seeds!)

Finally, you might be interested in a review about a common spice, curcumin (Hesari, et al., 2019).

# References

Al-Saleh, I., & Al-Enazi, S. (2011). Trace metals in lipsticks.

*Toxicological & Environmental Chemistry, 93,* 1149-1165.

Blakey, K., et al. (2014). Is fluoride a risk factor for bone cancer? Small area analysis of osteosarcoma and Ewing sarcoma diagnosed among 9-49-year-olds in Great Britain, 1980-2005.

*International Journal of Epidemiology, 43*(1), 224-234.

Davidson, K., et al. (2016). Microplastic ingestion by wild and cultured Manila clams (Venerupis philippinarum) from Baynes Sound, British Columbia.

*Archives of Environmental Contamination and Toxicology, 71*(2), 147156, and following.

Frostegård, J., et al. (2007). Atheroprotective natural anti-phosphorylcholine antibodies of IgM subclass are decreased in Swedish controls as compared to non-westernized individuals from New Guinea.

*Nutrition & Metabolism (London), 4,* 7 and following.

[**Note:** These researchers found higher levels of IgM-antibodies

**against phosphorylcholine in the population in Kitava, New Guinea with a traditional lifestyle, compared to Swedish control subjects.]**

Harpaz, T., et al. (2018). The effect of ethanol on telomere dynamics and regulation in human cells.

*Cells, 7*(10), 169 and following.

[ Note: Telomeres protect chromosome ends from chromosomal fusion and degradation, and thus confer genomic stability; **they also play a role in cellular aging and disease. Furthermore, environmental, physiological, and even mental stress can adversely affect telomere function in humans! This study shows that moderate consumption of alcohol ("social drinking") is a stress that can increase the risk of getting cancer!**]

Harrison, P.T.C. (2005). Review. Fluoride in water: A UK perspective.

*Journal of Fluorine Chemistry, 126* (11-12), 1448-1456.

Hesari, A., et al. (2019). Chemopreventive and therapeutic potential of curcumin in esophageal cancer: Current and future status.

*International Journal of Cancer, 144*(6), 1215-1226.

Kulshreshtha, S., et al. (February 22, 2011). Handmade paper and cardboard industries: In health perspectives.

*Toxicology and Industrial Health, 27*(6), 515-521.

Lantz, P.M., et al. (2013). Radon, smoking, and lung cancer: The need to refocus radon control policy.

*American Journal of Public Health, 103*(3), 443-447.

Lindeberg, S., et al. (1994). Cardiovascular risk factors in a Melanesian population apparently free from stroke and ischaemic heart disease: The Kitava study.

*Journal of Internal Medicine, 236*(3), 331-340.

[Note: **As to why this population in Papua New Guinea was free of deaths due to strokes and ischemic heart disease, the authors point to their <u>not being overweight, low blood pressure, and healthy nutrition</u>!**]

Lucová, M., et al. (2013). Absorption of triphenylmethane dyes Brilliant Blue and Patent Blue through intact skin, shaven skin and lingual mucosa from daily life products.

*Food and Chemical Toxicology, 52*, 19-27.

Moghaddam, V.K., et al. (2018). High concentrations of fluoride can be increased risk of abortion.

*Biological Trace Elements Research, 185*(2), 262-265.

News Release, (February 19, 2013). Effects of human exposure to

hormone-disrupting chemicals examined in landmark report. World Health Organization, citing: "State of the Science of

Endocrine Disrupting Chemicals," a report by

*The United Nations Environment Programme (UNEP)* and *World Health Organization.*

Platzek, T. (2010). Risk from exposure to arylamines from consumer products and hair dyes.

*Frontiers in Bioscience E2,* 1169-1183.

Rarau, P., et al. (2017). Prevalence of non-communicable disease risk factors in three sites across Papua New Guinea: A cross-sectional study.

*BMJ Global Health, 2*(2), e000221 and following.

[Note: In this study, inhabitants of 3 geographically separated areas of Papua New Guinea were examined for risk factors for noncommunicable diseases. These risk factors, which varied widely among the respective inhabitants of the 3 areas, included **obesity, alcohol consumption, smoking, high blood pressure, physical inactivity, high cholesterol, and low HDL cholesterol.**]

Sharma, S., et al. (2017). Microplastic pollution, a threat to marine ecosystem and human health: A short review.

*Environmental Science and Pollution Research, 24*(27), 21539-21547.

Tohyama, E. (1996). Relationship between fluoride concentration in drinking water and mortality rate from uterine cancer in Okinawa Prefecture, Japan.

*Journal of Epidemiology, 6*(4), 184-191.

# APPENDIX 1.

# Diving Deeper

―――――――――― ★ ★ ★ ――――――――――

One of the purposes of this appendix is to provide a few (not exhaustive) sources of information for those who wish to "dive deeper" into the research literature on cancer. I feel that this is necessary because of the freedom of speech that allows us to say virtually anything we want – as long as no one is injured. The problem is that of "separating the wheat from the chaff" about the topics covered in this book. Many individuals have deceiving letters after their names, such as MD, PhD, MA, RD, etc.; though these are potentially impressive, they are deceiving when the individuals do not fully know (do not fully keep up with) the state-of-the-art in the various areas outlined in this book! There are many thousands of such "problems" on the Internet, in books, on blogs, on TV, etc.

Below, I list a few individuals whom I consider to be highly reliable. Whenever you read something in the health field that you think might need to be "fact checked," just compare it with the teachings of the following:

- William W. Li, MD (and DrWilliamLi.com)

- Sophia Lunt, PhD

- Vincent Li, MD

- Gabe Mirkin, MD (and DrMirkin.com, where you can sign up for his free weekly ezine). Doctor Mirkin scours the roughly 1,100 biomedical research journals, and shares his "take" on the articles he cites. He is known for having at least one relevant citation for virtually everything that he recommends!

The second purpose of this appendix is to share tools that I have found helpful in my work in the health field.

- **PubMed** is a free site created by the National Institutes of Health. This site allows searching for research publications by journal name, author, article title, similar topics, etc. In addition, it features references that cite a given research article; this powerful feature can quickly expand one's list of relevant research publications! One if its features is labelled the "Single Citation Matcher."

- **Google Scholar** (scholar.google.com) allows users to search a broader range of references, such as magazines, patents, etc.

# APPENDIX 2.

# A Typically Meal

---

**Brunch**

1. one large banana

2. around two or three servings of a bean dish (as a source of protein, etc.) served over a bed of true whole grains, such as quinoa, teff, wild rice (an "honorary grain"; actually, a grass), oat groats, etc. [Keep in mind that **most (if not all) brown rice is NOT a true whole grain; it has been processed to remove the nutritious outer husk! If it were a true whole grain, its contents of protein and fiber would be those of wild rice!**]

3. fresh, rinsed blueberries (about 2 servings)

4. two medium handfuls of cashew nuts (about 2 serving/2 ounces)

5. six dried dates

6. a medium handful of blackberries, about 1.5 servings

# CANCER

**Dinner**

- two or so servings of a bean dish (the same bean dish as for brunch, or, preferably, a different one) on a bed of true whole grains, such as quinoa or wild rice
- a total of three to four medium handfuls of nuts, divided between pistachios and cocktail peanuts
- fresh, rinsed red seedless grapes, about 2 servings
- sometimes one or two servings of guacamole

# APPENDIX 3.

## Getting your vegetables
### The easy way!

★ ★ ★

Some years ago, I realized that – although I was eating plenty of fruits, nuts, and protein, I was not getting enough vegetables. So, I created a recipe that would cure this deficiency!

I start with five or more veggies (frozen or fresh) that are available at my grocery store, such as green beans, broccoli, frozen riced cauliflower, squash, etc. Then, I add two or three sliced portabella mushrooms (which have aromatase inhibitors that fight cancers – among many other healthy phytochemicals), kale or spinach, one or two large red bell peppers, and one or two large red onions. **[Note: All of these vegetables are loaded with cancer-fighting and cancer-preventing phytochemicals, as is true of virtually all vegetables!]**

In a two-quart pot, I add three or four cups of water, and bring it to a boil. Then, I add the above vegetables, and bring the mixture to a boil again for seven to ten minutes. Next, I put this concoction – pot and all – into the freezer for cooling, for an hour or two, after which I pour the veggie mix into a plastic storage container, and thence into the refrigerator.

I prefer to eat this veggie mix without any seasonings, except salt, which I add just before eating it. However, suit yourself with whatever seasonings your taste buds prefer, and whether you add them during cooking or at time of eating; the sky is the limit for your choices and preferences! Also, obviously, choose vegetables which you enjoy best! – As noted above, most vegetables are nutrient-rich; however, there are exceptions, such as iceberg lettuce, which has virtually no major nutritional value, other than fiber.

## ENJOY!

# APPENDIX 4.

# CT Scans Can Greatly Increase the Risk for Cancers!

★ ★ ★

Doctors often order CT (Computed Tomography) scans to help diagnose any of a huge range of possible medical conditions. Sometimes CT scans are necessary, and sometimes they may not be necessary!

The problem with CT scans is that they cause a large amount of radiation to be inflicted on a patient's body, which can greatly increase their risks for cancers and other negative conditions. In the alternative, when a physician orders a CT scan, the patient should ask if an MRI (Magnetic Resonance Imaging) scan could suffice. **A CT scan can emit a radiation dosage up to <u>500 times greater than an MRI scan</u>!**

# APPENDIX 5.

# CANCER: Fact versus Fiction
## What YOU Need to Know

---------- ★ ★ ★ ----------

False: Most people believe that cancer is usually caused by <u>BAD GENETICS</u>.

<u>The Truth</u>: Only <u>5 to 10%</u> of cancers are caused by bad genetics.

<u>The Truth</u>: The other <u>90 to 95%</u> of cancers are caused by <u>ENVIRONMENTAL FACTORS</u> (for example, air pollution, cigarette smoke, "new-car smell," gasoline fumes, fumes from photocopy machines, new flooring from China, etc.), as well as the following:

<u>The Truth</u>: Poor or imperfect <u>NUTRITION</u>.

<u>The Truth</u>: Lack of a sufficient quantity of sufficiently demanding <u>EXERCISE</u> – *both* cardio exercise *and* strength-building exercises.

<u>The Truth</u>: An insufficient quantity of *deep* <u>SLEEP</u> virtually every night.

<u>The Truth</u>: Thus, based on the above, cancer usually is caused by

impairment of a person's <u>IMMUNE SYSTEM</u>! <u>Every one</u> of the above factors impacts the immune system!

# Reference

Mirkin, Gabe. (June 10, 2021.) Routine CT scans can increase cancer risk. *Mirkin Fitness & Health Newsletter.* [at DrMirkin.com. Gabe Mirkin, M.D. Free newsletter].

# DOC'S CREDENTIALS

---  ★ ★ ★  ---

When Doc Wilson's mother died from a kind of cancer that, at the time, was considered "incurable," he vowed to learn everything he could about causes, preventions, and cures for the common cancers. Subsequently, Doc was also diagnosed with cancer – even though he had led a close-to-exemplary lifestyle with respect to nutrition, exercise, sleep, and stress. Doc then decided to share his story and his illuminating findings about cancer through a book, as well as through seminars, and one-on-one and group health consultations.

Doc Wilson's ground-breaking book, ***CANCER. Causes, Preventions, Cures. What the Food and Beverage Does NOT Want You to Know!*** addresses critically needed information that is not readily available from most members of the medical community. As is implied in the book's subtitle, the food and beverage industry is not in the business of educating the public about cutting-edge research that has the potential not only to help some cancer patients cure their cancers, but also to at least reduce anxiety levels, and even cancer levels, in other patients when they follow Doc's prescriptions! Of course, since we live in a capitalistic society, we should not expect Food and Beverage entities to spend time and money on undercutting their respective, money-generating businesses; hence the need for <u>an unbiased "outsider"</u> like Doc.

Doc's extensive background in biomedical sciences, and experience as a Personal Trainer and as a medical school professor, have provided Doc with a varied, rich, and relevant foundation for writing *CANCER*.

### **Brief Summary of Doc's Technical Training:**

- B.A. (Biology, Chemistry), Kalamazoo College, Kalamazoo, MI. Included Foreign Study: 6 months, University of Strasbourg, France.

- M.A. (Physiology), SUNY at Buffalo, "Passed with Distinction." NY.

- Ph.D. (Physiology, Biochemistry), University of Illinois at Urbana.

- Postdoctoral Fellowship (Biochemistry, Physical Chemistry), Duke University, Durham, NC.

- University of Maryland School of Medicine, Founder & Director, Renal Laboratory, Baltimore, MD.

Made in the USA
Middletown, DE
24 September 2023